A PATIENT'S GUIDE TO

CANCER CARE

FIGHTING CANCER BODY, MIND & SPIRIT

VIRGINIA B. MORRIS
SOPHIE FORRESTER

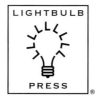

LIGHTBULB

PRESS ®

LIGHTBULB PRESS
Project Team

Lead Writer and Researcher Bess Newman
Editorial Staff Rachel Baumgartner, Joan Kim, Starr Marcello, Karen Halloran Meldrom, Mavis Morris, Tania Sanchez

Design Director Dave Wilder
Design Mercedes Feliciano
Production and Illustration Kara W. Hatch, Terry Marks, Katharina Menner, Tina Sbrigato, Thomas F. Trojan

SPECIAL THANKS

First, to all the cancer patients who have challenged and continue to challenge this disease at every turn, and have thus created the body of knowledge that is outlined in this book.

Second, to several members of the finest group of cancer patient care experts who contributed to this book in their quest to offer helpful options to those patients and their caregivers:

Lise Alschuler, ND; Tim Birdsall, ND; Elizabeth Crane, MEd, MBA; Bernard Eden, MD; Karen Gilbert, RPT; Christine Girard, ND; Doug Kelly, MD; Carolyn Lammersfeld, MS, RD, LD; Rev. Michael Langham; Stan Maravilla, RPT; Julie Martin, ND; Kathy McCauley, RD; Rev. Percy McCray; Jack Moore; Nora Orrick; Katherine Puckett, PhD; and Sybilann Williams, MD.

And, to a true visionary, Richard J Stephenson, who following the tragic loss of his mother, Mary Brown Stephenson, to this disease, has dedicated so much of his life, and created enormous passion in many others, to win the war against cancer.

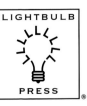

*W*e're all touched by cancer at some point during our lives, some of us personally, and others through the experience of a family member, friend, or coworker. In addition, cancer rates are on the rise around the world. In the US alone, almost one and a half million people are diagnosed with the disease every year.

For everyone who has been affected by cancer, the experience drives a powerful quest for information. Information and knowledge are empowering tools in the hands of cancer patients and their loved ones, giving them the confidence to seek treatment and support that meets their physical, emotional, and spiritual needs.

The challenge today is not finding information, but distilling it. In fact, many of our patients liken their quest for information to trying to drink from a fire hose. They're simply overwhelmed by the volume. In this book, working with our partners at Lightbulb Press, we have tried to put an adjustable nozzle on that hose. We hope that *A Patient's Guide to Cancer Care* will allow you to find helpful information easily, and that the information you find will empower you to seek answers relevant to your own interests, experience, philosophies, and beliefs.

Armed with the knowledge that you can fight cancer on all fronts—body, mind, and spirit—we also hope you will find the right path to victory. We wish you great success, and welcome your thoughts and suggestions for improved information and treatment alternatives.

Stephen B. Bonner, President and CEO
Cancer Treatment Centers of America
Steve.bonner@ctca-corp.com
1-800-For-Help

A PATIENT'S GUIDE TO CANCER CARE

Treating the Whole Person

Enlist the forces of mind, body, and spirit to energize the process of healing.

If you or a loved one has been diagnosed with cancer, chances are you want to use every resource at your disposal to overcome it. That means working with a wide range of specialists who can help you make informed decisions about your treatment, and who support you on a variety of fronts—medical, nutritional, physical, psychological, and spiritual.

Just sorting through the information can be intimidating. There's so much to learn, and you want to make the best decisions. How do you know what applies to your situation, and what doesn't? You may have conflicting information from different care providers and sources. Whose information and judgment can you trust?

Your oncologist may have talked to you about conventional treatment options, such as radiation, chemotherapy, or surgery. But perhaps there are other approaches you want to explore, such as nutrition or naturopathic medicine. Maybe you've tried to discuss these with your oncologist or primary care physician (PCP). Even if they are supportive, chances are they're not in communication with a naturopathic physician about your treatment. So you may feel torn or pulled in different directions.

AN INDIVIDUAL APPROACH
Finding the right healthcare facility and care providers may be one of the first and most challenging steps in your treatment. It's important to seek out care providers who work in concert with treatment specialists in other disciplines to develop an individualized, multi-faceted treatment plan that's designed for you. Doing so can give you the best chance of recovery and

> **❝** Cancer affects every aspect of a person's life, so in the healing process it's important to take care of the whole person: mind, body, and spirit. **❞**
> Katherine L. Puckett, LCSW

the confidence of knowing that you and your caregivers are doing everything possible to overcome your cancer.

A WHOLE SPEC

Conventional

- Surgery
- Chemotherapy
- Radiation
- Immunotherapy
- Stem cell transplant

A POTENT COMBINATION
Conventional cancer treatments, such as surgery, radiation, and chemotherapy, are an important part of the treatment plans of many cancer patients. Not only have these approaches been used effectively for years. New techniques continue to evolve, making conventional cancer therapies safer, more effective, and less invasive all the time.

There's also plenty of evidence to suggest that augmenting conventional treatment with complementary therapies, such as nutrition and counseling, helps cancer patients tolerate and respond to treatment better and enjoy an enhanced quality of life. That's because good health and wellbeing help make your immune system stronger. And your immune system is your first line of defense in preventing, treating, and beating cancer.

ONE SIZE DOESN'T FIT ALL

Some complementary therapies help improve your overall health. Others work in individual, tumor-specific, treatment-specific ways to fight a particular type of cancer. Or they may work together with a specific conventional treatment to enchance its effectiveness, or relieve a certain side effect.

For instance, green tea has been found to increase the effectiveness of doxorubicin, a widely used chemotherapy drug. On the other hand, patients receiving cisplatin-, carboplatin-, or oxaliplatin-based chemotherapy may respond well to the herbs ginkgo biloba and milk thistle. And patients undergoing radiation therapy may benefit from vitamin A and niacinamide supplements.

M OF HEALING THERAPIES

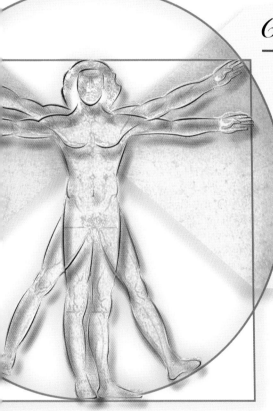

Complementary

- Naturopathic medicine
- Nutrition
- Exercise
- Mind-Body medicine
- Spiritual support
- Physical therapy
- Pain management

TO LEARN MORE
Comprehensive Cancer Care: Integrating Alternative, Complementary, and Conventional Therapies
by James S. Gordon, MD and Sharon Curtin, 2000

THE FULL COMPLEMENT

There are a wide variety of complementary therapies for you to consider that have been used successfully in cancer treatment. Among them:

Nutrition: A healthful, varied diet can help prevent many types of cancer, improve your response to treatment, and bolster your immune system.

Natural medicine: Naturopathic physicians use foods, supplements, plant-based substances, and a wide variety of traditional and experimental therapies to complement conventional treatment and to help restore the body's natural ability to heal itself.

Mind-Body medicine: Counseling, stress management, meditation, and other techniques can help you respond in the most effective way to your illness.

Spiritual support: Patients who nurture their spiritual side often feel better and experience less loneliness and fear during treatment.

Exercise and physical therapy: Moderate exercise and physical rehabilitation can help reduce the risk of cancer, promote recovery by stimulating your body's natural healing ability, and enhance the quality of your life.

Lives of a Cancer Cell

Understanding cancer makes it a less formidable opponent.

Many people tend to think of cancer as one disease. But the word **cancer** describes a large group of diseases that have certain traits in common, yet exhibit distinctive characteristics. In fact, there are over 200 known types of cancers that all behave in different ways, grow at different rates, and respond to different types of treatment. But what all types of cancer have in common is the growth of abnormal cells in the body that replicate rapidly, are difficult to destroy, and can overwhelm normal, healthy cells.

CELLS BY THE NUMBERS

Like all living organisms, your body consists of cells. The average human body is made up of about 60 trillion cells. Every day these cells divide billions of times, replacing worn out or damaged cells in an orderly, regulated way.

Out of all the billions of cells that your body creates each day, it's no wonder that it makes mistakes from time to time and creates abnormal cells. Usually your immune system recognizes these cells and repairs or eliminates them. In fact, many researchers believe that everyone develops pre-cancerous cells during his or her lifetime, yet less than half the population ever develops cancer.

WHY ME?

Why do some people develop cancer while others don't? Researchers are still trying to answer this question.

Cancer develops when DNA gets damaged. DNA is the primary

> **"**Cancer is rarely caused by a single factor; rather it is the result of a complex interaction between carcinogens, or cancer-causing substances in the environment, and heredity.**"**
> American Institute for Cancer Research

CONTRIBUTING FACTORS

- Medical history
- Hormonal influences
- Diet and nutrition
- Environment
- Lifestyle
- Past medical treatment

Genetic factors contribute to 15% of all cancers

Cancer cells divide in a rapid and disorderly way.

genetic material inside every cell that influences everything it does. If damaged cells are not repaired by the body, they become cancerous.

DNA can become damaged in a variety of ways and increase your risk of cancer. Some people may inherit damaged DNA genetically, making it more likely that they will develop certain types of cancer. Genetic irregularities are responsible for about 15% of all cancers. The other 85% are caused by environmental and lifestyle factors that you may or may not be able to control. For instance, healthy cells can become damaged because of poor dietary habits, smoking, or a sedentary lifestyle. Environmental factors, such as poor air quality, secondhand smoke, or exposure to carcinogens at work can raise your risk. Even living in an urban environment can increase the likelihood of developing cancer.

The good news is that whether or not your risk for cancer is inherited, making positive lifestyle changes can

Can lifestyle choices affect your risk of developing cancer? They sure can. For instance, smokers are ten times—or 1,000%—more likely to develop lung cancer than people who have never smoked.

PREVENTIVE ACTIONS

- Don't smoke
- Eat well
- Exercise
- Avoid pollution

A FORMIDABLE OPPONENT

Cancerous cells have certain properties that make them especially difficult for your body's immune system and other protective mechanisms to detect and destroy:

- Cancer cells can disguise themselves to become undetectable to your immune system
- Cancer cells grow in a rapid and disorderly way
- Cancer cells are not programmed to die like regular cells
- Cancer can **metastasize**, or spread, through the lymphatic system or the blood stream to another part of the body, creating multiple tumors
- Cancer cells can mutate, making them resistant to chemotherapy and radiation
- As cancer proliferates throughout the body, it can overwhelm the immune system and other functions, causing secondary infections and organ failure

reduce your chances of developing the disease. If you've been diagnosed, making healthy lifestyle choices can help you live longer—and feel better.

TOXIC OVERLOAD

Many researchers believe that the prevalence of cancer today is due to exposure to toxins in the environment, such as air pollution. Additives, pesticides, and artificial hormones in food also play a role. These toxins can damage your cellular structure, impair your immune system, and overtax your body's natural ability to rid itself of poisons and waste products. Even the stresses of modern life may affect your health.

You may be able to counteract your exposure to toxins by following a healthy lifestyle and strengthening your body's natural ability to heal itself.

- If you're a smoker, quit smoking.
- Choose whole, unprocessed, and organic foods. Wash all produce thoroughly.
- Exercise moderately if you're up to it. Exercise stimulates immune system function and your body's natural cleansing abilities.
- Reduce your stress level by getting enough rest and finding ways to relax.

AN AGE-OLD FOE

Cancer has afflicted people since the beginning of recorded history. Malignant tumors have been found in mummies and fossilized bones, and have been documented in ancient manuscripts.

According to tradition, the term **cancer** was coined by the Greek physician Hippocrates (460-370 BC). He used the word **carcinoma**, which means **crab** in Greek, probably because the swollen blood vessels surrounding a tumor were thought to look like crabs' legs.

Today, the word **carcinoma** is still used to describe the most common type of cancer. The more generic term, **cancer**, comes from the Latin word for crab.

TO LEARN MORE
www.cancerquest.org
Emory University website on cancer cell biology

Your Diagnosis

Take charge of your treatment and create a plan of action.

No one wants to be diagnosed with cancer. Whether you hear the news for the first time, or you're told that your cancer has spread or recurred, you may feel you've lost control of your life.

But in fact, the outlook has never been better for people with cancer. There are over nine million cancer survivors in the US, and new treatments are developed every week. Genetic research and other scientific advances continue to yield new clues into the causes of cancer, and how it can be overcome. Many types of cancer that were considered untreatable even ten years ago can now be managed effectively.

It's natural to feel depressed, angry, or hopeless after your diagnosis. But it's important to remember that as long as you're fighting, there's hope. People have recovered from virtually every type of cancer. Most cancer survivors agree that getting over your initial disbelief and dread is one of the hardest parts of the battle. They also agree that the most effective way to deal with your new situation is to take charge of all the information you're given and turn it into a plan of action.

DIAGNOSTIC TESTS

Doctors use a number of different methods to determine if you have cancer. In fact, since the initial symptoms can be vague or inconclusive, they often rely on a combination of exams. Your doctor may also use these tests during or after treatment to determine how effectively it's working.

 Blood tests can detect substances that are produced by certain cancers

 Scans such as mammograms, computed tomography (CT) scans, and magnetic resonance imaging (MRI) use radiation or magnetic waves to create pictures of internal organs

 Endoscopes use a small camera to see inside the body

Biopsies are the surgical removal of tissue for examination under a microscope

You'll want to ask your doctor which tests were performed, and why they indicate cancer. Some tests, or combination of tests, are more conclusive than others.

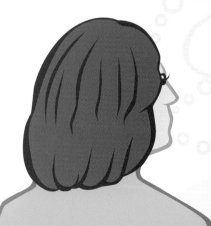

What's the latest research on my type of cancer?

Where should I go for a second opinion?

Where can I go for the latest treatment?

> **❝** *Most people who face cancer learn that the battle is as much a mental battle as it is a physical one. For many, greater knowledge about their disease, treatment choices, and prognosis can boost their capacities to handle any setbacks.* **❞**
>
> Harmon J. Eyre, MD,
> Dianne Partie Lange, and
> Lois B. Morris, *Informed Decisions*

How can I beat my cancer?

What's my plan of action?

How can family and friends help me through this?

Where can I talk to others who have survived my type of cancer?

THE GAMUT OF EMOTIONS

People who are diagnosed with cancer may go through a period of denial about their illness. They may be angry and not recognize the real cause of their rage. They may feel depressed or frustrated, and have trouble responding to family members and friends. These feelings are perfectly natural and may occur at different times and in different combinations.

A cancer diagnosis may be a traumatic event, and the emotional reaction is different for every patient. Don't let anyone tell you how to feel or rush you toward acceptance. Dealing with your emotions at your own pace is the best way to move ahead.

CANCER STATISTICS

One of the first questions many patients ask their doctors is, *How much time do I have?* But no one can tell you how long you will live, or how well you will respond to treatment. The only information a doctor can give you is the statistical average for a large and diverse group of people with a similar diagnosis.

If you ask for this information, your doctor will probably tell you the **five-year survival rate**—the percentage of patients who are cancer-free after five years.

But keep in mind that these statistics include patients who had other health problems, and patients who refused all treatment. These numbers are also based on patients treated 10 or 20 years ago, without today's advanced therapies. In fact, recent studies indicate that widely cited cancer survival statistics may be too pessimistic. In other words, survival rates may be inaccurate and misleading, and since statistics apply to groups, not individuals, they don't translate into a personal prognosis.

Many experts feel that time limits can become a self-fulfilling prophecy. They recommend that you ask instead what you can do to fight the cancer and maximize your odds by working with the best doctors and getting access to the latest technology. Countless patients who were told they wouldn't make it are still alive today.

DO YOUR HOMEWORK

For most cancer patients, there's no medical reason to rush into treatment, so it's a good idea to take time and learn your options.

1 Learn the exact type and stage of your cancer.

2 Get a second opinion. An accurate diagnosis is crucial to effective treatment, so you want either confirmation or a new perspective to pursue.

3 Call the NCI's Cancer Information Service at 800-4-CANCER for the latest information and treatments for your type of cancer.

4 Keep a copy of all your medical records and test results in case you decide to change doctors or hospitals, or seek additional opinions.

The Language of Cancer

Words are powerful decision-making tools.

Breast cancer survivor and patient advocate Vickie Girard likens a cancer diagnosis to waking up in a foreign country, where you don't know the language and customs, and you have no maps to find your way home.

In the first weeks after your diagnosis, you'll encounter an array of specialists, tests, treatments, terminology, and decisions. Understanding the essentials of your diagnosis can help you gain control of your situation and make informed decisions about your treatment.

TYPES OF CANCER

Your treatment begins with an accurate and thorough diagnosis. By defining all the characteristics of the cancer, your doctors can predict how it's likely to progress and tailor treatments to take advantage of its vulnerabilities.

There are four major types of cancer, based on the type of tissue where the tumor originates:

Carcinomas occur on the skin and in the layer of tissue that lines the body's internal surfaces. There are two kinds of carcinomas: **adenocarcinomas** that start in the cells covering a gland, such as the thyroid, and **squamous cell carcinomas** that form in the cells covering other internal tissues, such as the cervix or lungs. 80% of tumors are classified as carcinomas.

Sarcomas start in connective tissue such as muscle, fat, cartilage, and bone. Tumors in fatty tissue are called **liposarcomas**, and bone tumors are called **osteosarcomas**.

Leukemias are **hematologic**, or blood, cancers that originate in the blood or blood-forming organs. These cancer cells don't usually form solid tumors.

Lymphomas are hematologic cancers that develop in the lymphatic system—the network of nodes and vessels that transports nutrients through the body.

Since most parts of the body are composed of different kinds of tissue, it's possible for two patients with tumors of the same primary site to have different types of cancer. Uterine cancers, for example, are usually carcinomas, but they can also occur as sarcomas, if they develop in the connective tissue of the uterus.

> **TO LEARN MORE**
> *The Complete Cancer Survival Guide*
> by Peter Teeley and Philip Bashe, 2000

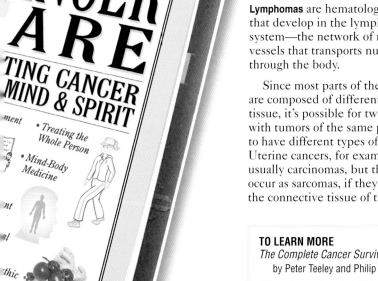

LIGHTBULB ☼ PRESS®

PATIENT'S GUIDE TO
ANCER
ARE

TING CANCER
MIND & SPIRIT

• *Treating the Whole Person*

• *Mind-Body Medicine*

OPHIE FORREST

> **“** *Treating cancer properly depends on defining each and every tumor very precisely.* **”**
>
> Malin Dollinger, MD,
> Ernest H. Rosenbaum, MD, and
> Greg Cable, *Everyone's Guide to Cancer Therapy*

STAGING

The **stage** of your cancer is a measure of whether and how far it has spread. Your doctor might take samples of your lymph nodes to test them for cancerous cells, and determine the stage of the disease.

The stages range from one to four, with lower stages indicating little or no spreading. Higher stages may mean the cancer has spread from the original site to distant tissues and might need more aggressive therapy.

When cancer cells **metastasize**, they break off from the primary tumor and circulate through the lymph system or blood to resettle in other parts of the body.

MAKING THE GRADE

The grade of your cancer is a measure of how closely its cells resemble normal cells. A pathologist examines a sample of your cancerous cells to determine their grade. A low-grade cancer—grade one or two—has cells that are similar in appearance to normal cells. A high-grade cancer—grade three or four—contains cells that look very different from healthy cells. In general, low-grade cancers are less aggressive and respond better to treatment than high-grade cancers.

The staging and grading process is important because it helps your doctors determine how to treat your cancer most effectively.

TUMOR MARKERS

Certain kinds of cancers release proteins, hormones, and other substances into your blood, or cause your body to produce certain substances called **tumor markers**. By testing your blood to measure the levels of these tumor markers, doctors are able to diagnose and track cancer. For instance, high levels of **prostate specific antigen (PSA)** might indicate prostate cancer.

Tumor markers are also tracked during treatment. Falling PSA levels, for example, might confirm that therapies have been effective. Other tumor markers include CA-125 for ovarian cancer, AFP for liver cancer, CA 15-3 and CA 27-29 for breast cancer, and CEA and CA-19 for colorectal and other cancers. Not all cancers correlate to tumor markers, but it's worth asking your oncologist if tumor markers can help you track your illness.

PSA

CA-125

AFP

CA-153

CA 27-29

CEA

CA-19

LEARN THE LANGUAGE

Primary tumor. A cancer is named after its primary site, or the part of the body in which it develops. For instance, cancer that develops in the breast and spreads to the bone is still called breast cancer, not bone cancer.

Metastasis. When cancer spreads from the primary site to other organs or tissues of the body, it is said to metastasize. Cancer usually spreads through the blood or the lymphatic system.

Remission. When diagnostic tests show that cancer is no longer present, the cancer is in remission. Some doctors use this term and **NED** (no evidence of disease) interchangeably. While cancer cells may remain, they're undetectable.

Recurrence. The return of cancer after a time of remission.

Pathologist. A medical doctor who specializes in diagnosing diseases by examining samples of tissue, blood, and body fluids.

*P*reparing for Treatment

Give yourself the best chance to win the fight against cancer.

You may feel that the success of your cancer treatment is completely in the hands of your doctors and other health professionals. That's not the case. There's a lot you can do to put yourself in a stronger position to benefit from therapy, tolerate treatment better, and recover more quickly—even if this isn't your first battle with cancer.

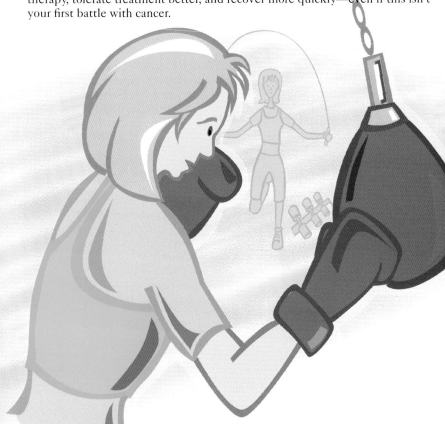

FORTIFY FOR THE FIGHT

Some patients liken their fight against cancer to training for the Olympics. Like an athlete, you want to make sure that your body is in peak form for the challenges ahead. While staying in shape may sound like a tall order when you've got cancer, it's an effective way to contribute to the success of your treatment.

Eating a wholesome, nutrient-rich diet, getting enough rest and relaxation, and staying as physically active as you are able will make you feel healthier and more confident about your treatment. Doing so may also help make your treatment more effective because your immune system will be strengthened.

And if you establish good habits before you get started, you'll also be more likely to continue your healthy routines once treatment begins.

> **❝** *If you've been eating a healthy diet, you'll go into treatment with reserves to help keep up your strength, prevent body tissue from breaking down, rebuild tissue, and maintain your defenses against infection.* **❞**
> National Cancer Institute

SET UP A SUPPORT SYSTEM

Your network of friends, family, community, and fellow cancer patients can be an indis-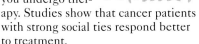pensable source of encouragement, inspiration, and practical support as you undergo therapy. Studies show that cancer patients with strong social ties respond better to treatment.

It's smart to anticipate changes to your schedule ahead of time and enlist help. For instance, you might have to arrange a new work schedule, or ask a friend to take over some of your household chores, accompany you to appointments, or help out with childcare.

A support group of other cancer patients is also a great resource. People who've experienced cancer therapy firsthand can provide inspiration as well as practical advice.

GET INFORMED

Before you start treatment, ask the questions that are on your mind. Knowing what to expect can ease anxiety and help you prepare emotionally for treatment.

1 Ask if your doctor is going to measure how your cancer is responding at any point during treatment. That way, you'll have more information about how well the therapy is working.

2 Learn about all the possible side effects of your therapy. Chances are you won't experience them all, and most side effects are now manageable. But being prepared lets you create a plan for dealing with whatever comes your way.

3 Ask your doctor which symptoms or side effects might indicate a serious complication. Losing or gaining more than five pounds in a week, for example, should be reported to your doctor. Catching problems early can keep them from getting worse.

TO LEARN MORE
www.cancer.org
American Cancer Society website

PREPARING FOR SIDE EFFECTS

Some side effects are especially troubling. You'll want to have a game plan in place ahead of time:

Fatigue is a common side effect. Cancer-related fatigue is more intense than plain tiredness, and you may have to take frequent breaks, delegate chores, or plan regular naps into your schedule. Moderate exercise and good nutrition can boost your energy immensely.

Hair loss can be one of the most emotionally difficult side effects of chemotherapy. Many cancer survivors recommend that you buy a wig before you begin treatment. It can be worth investing in a good one, especially since your insurance may cover part of the cost. Others prefer scarves and baseball caps to wigs, which can be hot and itchy. Some patients shave their own heads at the first sign of hair loss, in order to be in control of the process.

Infertility is a risk with some cancers and cancer therapies. Talk to an oncologist, especially if you plan on having children after treatments are done. You may be able to preserve sperm or eggs before treatment to use in the future.

Sexual desire can change or diminish as a result of the physical and emotional aspects of treatment. Your oncologist may be able to recommend a counselor who can work with you and your partner.

VISIT THE DENTIST
It's a good idea to see your dentist before you start treatments. Chemo and radiation can cause tooth decay and make you more susceptible to gum and mouth infections. Taking care of any dental work ahead of time may prevent problems later on.

Conventional Therapies

For most people, conventional medicine is the cornerstone of treatment.

One of the first questions you probably asked after hearing your cancer diagnosis was, *How can I get better?* Most likely, your oncologist told you about conventional cancer treatments, including surgery, radiation, and chemotherapy. **Conventional therapies** are the foundation of most people's cancer treatment. They're based on established scientific principles and have been proven effective countless times.

In fact, one of the great advantages of conventional therapies is that scientists and doctors have had years to evaluate their effectiveness on a wide range of people and to continually refine the tools and techniques of treatment. Most important, conventional therapies have cured millions of people and have improved the outlook for millions more.

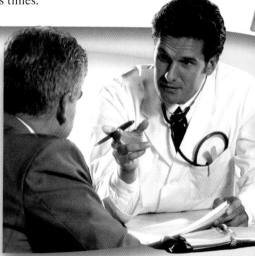

DIFFERENT PATHS TO HEALING

Sometimes conventional treatments are used to eliminate all traces of cancer or to prevent it from recurring. Other times they're used to help people manage the disease so that they can continue to lead fulfilling lives. While there is a wide range of conventional therapies, most—though not all—fall into one of the following categories:

Surgery—
an operation to remove part or all of a tumor

Chemotherapy—
prescription drugs that can debilitate or destroy cancer cells

Radiation—
energy that damages and destroys cancerous cells

Immunotherapy—
drugs and therapies that stimulate your immune system, helping your body fight cancer more effectively

You may receive one conventional therapy, or several—sometimes called **combination** or **multimodality treatment**. For instance, you might first receive radiation or chemotherapy to reduce the size of a tumor, and then undergo surgery to remove what remains.

Sometimes conventional therapies are combined: For example, you might receive radiation therapy during surgery, when the tumor is exposed and can be treated with a single high dose of radiation.

LEARN THE LANGUAGE

Depending on how they are used, most therapies can be local or systemic, primary or adjuvant.

- **Local** therapies treat the part of the body where the tumor is located.
- **Systemic** treatments work on your whole body. They are especially useful for cancers that may have spread.
- **Primary** therapies are the core of your cancer treatment. Many different therapies can work as primary treatment—it depends on your type of cancer.

> **❝** *Cancer treatment is improving—saving lives and extending survival for people with cancers at many sites.* **❞**
> National Cancer Institute 2001
> Cancer Progress Report

- **Adjuvant** treatments are used in addition to the primary therapy, to make it more powerful or reduce its side effects. **Neo-adjuvant** therapies take place before a primary treatment. They prepare your body so that the primary treatment will be more effective.

For example, you can receive chemotherapy locally, directly at the site of a tumor. More often, it is a systemic treatment that circulates throughout your body. Radiation may be the primary therapy for some cancers, but for others it is used as an adjuvant therapy before or after surgery.

A PERSONALIZED PRESCRIPTION

Even though a treatment is described as conventional, it doesn't mean that you should receive assembly-line care. Each person's situation is unique. Your doctor will consider your particular diagnosis, along with your medical history, age, and current health, when advising which course of treatment is best for you.

When learning about your options, it can help to remember that while some conventional therapies may have been traumatic for people in the past, advanced medical technologies have made many of them much easier to tolerate. New drugs and complementary therapies can relieve many side effects and help your body heal faster.

TEAMWORK

It's important that your oncologist and other caregivers, such as nutritionists and naturopathic doctors, are communicating about your treatment. By working together, they can give you the best chance of beating cancer.

TO LEARN MORE
Everyone's Guide to Cancer Therapy
by Malin Dollinger, MD,
Ernest H. Rosenbaum, MD, and
Greg Cable, 1998

BALANCING FORCES

Conventional therapies aren't the only weapons at your disposal. Increasingly, doctors and scientists are recognizing that good nutrition, exercise, and spiritual and emotional health play an important role in treating and preventing cancer. There are a number of healing philosophies outside of conventional medicine, including **Eastern** and **botanical** therapies, that can dramatically improve your wellbeing during treatment, and even help make your primary therapy more effective.

Ask your oncologist about other forms of treatment. If he or she can't provide the information you need, or is unhelpful, you may want to investigate integrative cancer care facilities that specialize in fighting cancer on a variety of fronts.

WATCHFUL WAITING

If you're older or have a slow-growing cancer, you may decide to watch and wait rather than immediately undertake aggressive conventional therapy. This means working closely with your healthcare team as you monitor your progress and using complementary therapies to build your immune system. While some experts advise this approach in certain circumstances, you'll also want to weigh all the possible risks.

Surgery

Modern surgery brings together ancient traditions and innovative techniques.

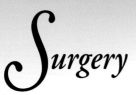

Surgery is one of the oldest, most effective, and most widely practiced medical arts. Surgeons remove appendixes, restore vision, and mend broken bones every day. And while surgery has been performed since the beginning of human civilization, new innovations and techniques continue to make surgery one of the most effective and versatile cancer treatments today.

About 60% of all cancer patients undergo a surgical procedure of some kind. While surgery is one of the most successful ways of curing contained tumors that haven't yet spread to other parts of the body, there are a variety of other ways surgery is used to help prevent, diagnose, and treat cancer:

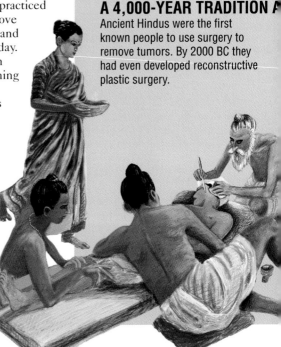

A 4,000-YEAR TRADITION A
Ancient Hindus were the first known people to use surgery to remove tumors. By 2000 BC they had even developed reconstructive plastic surgery.

- **Preventive** surgery removes precancerous, abnormal, and sometimes normal tissue that could become cancerous.

- **Diagnostic** surgery is used to detect whether a disease is present. In a **biopsy**, a small portion of tissue is removed to find out if it is cancerous.

- **Staging** surgery removes tissue to see how widespread the cancer is. The stage of your cancer will help doctors determine the best course of treatment.

- **Curative** surgery is the removal of a tumor that has not spread beyond its original site. Your doctor may prescribe chemotherapy or radiation after surgery to treat any cancerous cells that have been left behind.

- **Cytoreductive** or **debulking** surgery removes most of the tumor, but not the complete mass. Usually it's followed with chemotherapy

or radiation to destroy the rest of the cancer.

- **Palliative** surgery is performed to relieve cancer symptoms.

- **Reconstructive** surgery rebuilds tissue to restore the function or appearance of a part of the body that may have been affected by cancer or during treatment.

You may undergo different types of surgery during your treatment and recovery. Someone with breast cancer, for instance, might have a biopsy done to diagnose the cancer. Then the doctor might perform curative surgery to remove the tumor. Some months later, there may be reconstructive surgery to restore the appearance of the breast.

While surgery can sometimes be a traumatic experience, it offers the possibility of substantial relief and even cure for many people with cancer.

" Surgery offers the greatest chance for cure for many types of cancers. "
American Cancer Society

the sentinel nodes, doctors are able to remove far fewer lymph nodes for a biopsy, so patients experience reduced side effects and can expect a speedier recovery. Knowing the status of the sentinel nodes can help doctors more accurately determine the right course of treatment.

TODAY'S INNOVATIONS

Sentinel node biopsy

Ultrasonic surgical aspiration

Anesthesia machine

PIONEERING NEW METHODS

Innovations in technique are making surgery less invasive all the time, while improving the likelihood that your doctor can remove most or all of your cancer.

One such breakthrough is **ultrasonic surgical aspiration**. Sound waves are used to break the tumor into small fragments, which are then vacuumed away from the cancerous site. This treatment can effectively **debulk** tumors, and help doctors remove as much of the cancer as possible.

Another innovation is **sentinel node biopsy**, which helps doctors more accurately detect **metastatic** cancers using less invasive surgical techniques. Metastatic cancers are those that have spread from the primary site to nearby lymph nodes or other parts of the body. A procedure called **sentinel lymph node mapping** uses dyes or radioactive materials to help your doctors identify the first lymph nodes—called the sentinel nodes—where a metastatic cancer may spread. By identifying

CHECK THE MARGINS

During surgery to remove a tumor, your surgeon will also remove some of the tissue that borders the tumor, known as the **margin**. After the operation, a **pathologist** will examine this tissue under a microscope for signs of cancer cells. A **clear margin** shows no cancerous cells, and means it's likely that all the cancer was removed from the body. A **positive margin** contains cancer cells, and your doctor will recommend additional surgery or other conventional treatment. Even patients with clear margins might benefit from adjuvant therapies, since there's always a chance that undetected cancer cells remain after surgery.

AN INFORMED DECISION

Before your surgery, you'll be asked to sign a consent form. This is a legal document confirming that your doctor has fully explained the operation, its risks, and your other options. Before you agree, you'll want to confirm that surgery is the most appropriate treatment. For some cancers, such as prostate and breast, there may be a non-invasive alternative, such as high dose rate brachytherapy.

FEEL NO PAIN

One of the most important aspects of modern surgery, **anesthesia**, was developed by a physician named Crawford Long. In 1842, Dr. Long used ether to sedate a patient during the removal of a tumor. Today, anesthesiologists are doctors who specialize in sedation before surgery so that patients feel no pain during the operation. **Local anesthesia** and **regional anesthesia** numb portions of the body so that you may be awake during the procedure. Under **general anesthesia** you will be unconscious for the duration of the operation.

19

*C*hemotherapy

Anti-cancer drugs are potent prescriptions.

The idea of undergoing **chemotherapy**, or chemo, can sometimes seem as scary as a cancer diagnosis itself. Probably no form of cancer treatment provokes as much anxiety—or as much controversy. In fact, a few cancer patients refuse chemotherapy altogether because they fear the side effects and other health risks that can arise from treatment.

The term **chemotherapy** applies to a broad range of anti-cancer drugs that your doctor may prescribe in hundreds of different combinations and administer in many different ways. Just as a doctor prescribes specific antibiotics to treat an infection, your oncologist may prescribe a specific course of chemotherapy depending on your diagnosis.

GETTING BETTER ALL THE TIME

In some cases, new techniques such as **fractionated dose chemotherapy** may help make chemotherapy more effective while at the same time minimizing the side effects. Plus, there are a variety of medicines and natural therapies that may help you tolerate treatment better. For instance, certain medications can dramatically lessen the severity of nausea, a common side effect of chemotherapy. Some natural therapies may even help make some specific anti-cancer drugs more powerful.

Best of all, for many patients, chemotherapy is a proven strategy for treating—and beating—cancer.

HOW CHEMO WORKS

What chemotherapy drugs all have in common is the ability to destroy cancer cells. But cancer cells are not foreign organisms, like bacteria: They're damaged cells reproduced by your own body. That means that it's impossible to destroy cancer cells without affecting some of your healthy cells as well. And because chemotherapy targets cells that reproduce rapidly, like cancer cells, some of your normal cells that reproduce quickly may also be affected. For instance, the cells in your hair follicles, gastrointestinal tract, bone marrow, and mucous membranes normally reproduce quickly. That's why some cancer patients experience side effects such as hair loss, nausea, ulcers, and mouth sores during treatment.

The good news is that healthy cells can repair themselves faster than cancerous ones. Unlike cancer cells, which often lack internal repair mechanisms, normal cells that are damaged during chemotherapy can recover after your treatment is over.

AN IMPORTANT ALLY

About 75% of all cancer patients in the US receive chemotherapy. Your doctor may recommend it as the central part of your treatment plan or in combination with other conventional therapies, such as surgery and radiation. Depending on your diagnosis, you may receive chemotherapy to:

- Cure your cancer
- Reduce and control tumors
- Relieve pain or other symptoms you may be experiencing

You might receive chemotherapy over several weeks, several months, or possibly a year, and it may be administered at your doctor's office, in a hospital, or even at home. Most often chemo is given through an IV, although some receive it as an injection, or orally, as a pill or liquid. But no matter how or where you're treated, the administration of chemotherapy is almost never painful.

WEIGHING THE RISKS

Some cancer patients have misgivings about chemotherapy. Certain treatments have long-term risks, including heart and liver damage. Others may even increase your chances of developing other types of cancer. Sometimes, the treatment may seem worse than the disease itself.

It's important to investigate the specific type of chemotherapy your doctor is recommending. The kinds of side effects you may experience, and their severity, will depend on the drug, or drugs, you're taking, the dosage, and the duration of your treatment. For some patients, the side effects are minimal, while for others they may be significant.

As you explore your treatment options, you'll need to weigh the potential benefits against the potential risks with your doctors. But for most cancer patients, the biggest risk is going untreated.

One of the advantages of chemotherapy is that it is a systemic treatment that affects your entire body, attacking even undetected cancer cells.

What's more, side effects can almost always be successfully treated, so let your medical team know if you are uncomfortable or have an unpleasant reaction.

TO LEARN MORE
www.cancer.gov
National Cancer Institute website

NEW TECHNIQUES

New techniques are being developed all the time that help make chemotherapy more effective.

Fractionated dose chemotherapy. Your total dose is administered in small amounts over several days, rather than all at once, as with traditional chemotherapy. This may increase your overall exposure to medication while reducing side effects.

Intra-arterial chemotherapy (IAC). Used in the treatment of liver, head, face, neck, pancreatic, and pelvic cancers, IAC is the delivery of chemotherapy directly through an artery that leads to the site of a tumor. IAC may improve effectiveness while reducing the toxicity of treatment.

Intraperitoneal chemotherapy. This approach is used to treat ovarian cancer. Chemotherapy is administered directly to your peritoneal area, or abdominal cavity.

Chemotherapy sensitivity testing. Before treatment begins, there are several methods of evaluating which drugs will be more likely to work—and which will be less likely—in treating individual cancers. Test results showing that a particular approach has little chance of working can be especially valuable when there's a choice between two or more possible treatments.

TAILOR-MADE CHEMO

One state-of-the-art approach combines aspects of **chemotherapy** and **immunotherapy**. In some cases, the oncologist can match your cancer cells with laboratory-made antibodies, called **monoclonal antibodies**. These antibodies, once they are injected into the body, can recognize and attack the cancer cells.

A WINNER IN MORE WAYS THAN ONE
Chemotherapy doesn't always have to be debilitating. Four-time Tour de France winner Lance Armstrong biked 30 to 40 miles a day while undergoing chemotherapy. While that's a hard act to follow, many people are able to maintain their normal schedule throughout chemotherapy.

$\mathcal{R}$adiation Therapy

The power of radiation energizes the fight against cancer.

Over the past 30 years, radiation has developed into a highly sophisticated area of medicine. Combining radiation therapy with advances in physics, biology, and computer engineering, new techniques are being developed that improve the effectiveness of radiation while limiting its impact on healthy tissue. That means that people undergoing radiation therapy today often experience fewer side effects and have better results than they would have even five years ago.

> **TO LEARN MORE**
> *The Chemotherapy & Radiation Therapy Survival Guide*
> by Judith McKay, RN, and Nancee Hirano, RN, 1998

HOW RADIATION WORKS

Radiation is energy in the form of heat or light that travels through space. Sunlight is one of the many forms of radiation. X-rays that your doctors and dentists use during routine medical exams are another. In fact most natural substances—including your body's cells—contain measurable amounts of radiation.

In cancer therapy, high energy X-rays—similar to what your doctor or dentist uses, but much more powerful—are directed at your tumor. The radiation damages the DNA and other structural aspects of the cancer cells. This either kills the cells immediately or weakens them so that they cannot reproduce.

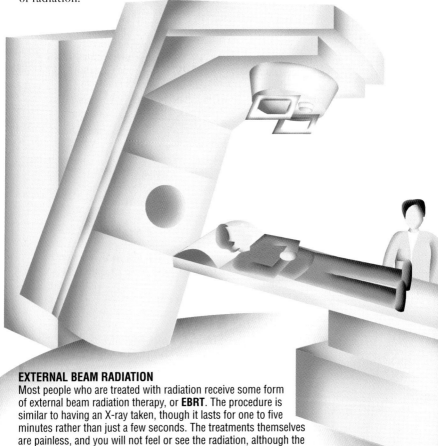

EXTERNAL BEAM RADIATION

Most people who are treated with radiation receive some form of external beam radiation therapy, or **EBRT**. The procedure is similar to having an X-ray taken, though it lasts for one to five minutes rather than just a few seconds. The treatments themselves are painless, and you will not feel or see the radiation, although the machine might make noise. People receiving external radiation are not radioactive, and pose no danger of exposing friends and family to radiation.

HEALING RAYS

About 60% of all people with cancer receive radiation therapy. Like other powerful treatments, it's administered in different ways to achieve different results:

- For some patients, radiation may be the main form of conventional treatment they receive to cure their cancer
- Radiation may be used before surgery or chemotherapy to shrink the size of a tumor
- Sometimes radiation is used after surgery or chemotherapy to eliminate any cancer cells that might remain
- Radiation may also be used to ease any pain caused by cancer

INTERNAL RADIATION THERAPY

Internal radiation, or **low dose rate brachytherapy**, is becoming an increasingly common procedure for people with localized tumors. It enables doctors to deliver high doses of radiation to a small area. During brachytherapy, the oncologist implants tiny radioactive wires or pellets very near or within the tumor. The implants may be permanent or temporary, although the permanent implants give off radiation for a few weeks or months at most, after which they become inactive.

You may need to stay in the hospital for up to a week to receive brachytherapy. During your stay, your visits with friends and family may be limited to protect them from unnecessary radiation exposure. Once you are released from the hospital, it's perfectly safe to be in contact with people.

CHOOSING A TREATMENT CENTER

If you're having radiation therapy, you'll want to find the best facility for the type of treatment you need.

> **❝** *Modern chemotherapy and radiation therapy are powerful and in many cases highly effective weapons in the fight against cancer.* **❞**
>
> Judith McKay, RN, and Nancee Hirano, RN, *The Chemotherapy & Radiation Therapy Survival Guide*

Radiation comes from atoms, the building blocks of matter. Everything that exists in the universe—planets, stars, minerals, plants, and all living things—consists of atoms. Most atoms are considered **stable**, which means that they remain constant, and that they can join together with other stable atoms to form molecules.

In the late 1800s, scientists discovered that a few atoms are **unstable**. Unstable atoms contain excess energy, which means that they may undergo a spontaneous change or reaction, releasing energy into the environment. Some of the energy that unstable atoms release is radiation.

It wasn't long before scientists found ways to harness radioactive energy and began exploring its effects on human cells. Among the pioneers in this field were Henri Becquerel, Wilhelm Roentgen, Pierre Curie, and Marie Curie, the two-time Nobel prize winner.

One of their early, important insights into radiation was that, while it could be damaging to healthy tissue in high doses, it was especially lethal to cancer cells. Scientists soon began treating people with skin cancer and other malignant tumors with radiation. The first case of a cure was reported in 1899.

Usually your choices are the outpatient department of a cancer center or hospital, or an independent clinic. The chief considerations are the sophistication of the radiation equipment and how convenient the facility is for you to reach.

State-of-the-art equipment provides more accurate radiation therapy. Many, but not all, facilities keep track of new advances and keep their machinery current.

Convenience is an issue because the radiation treatments are usually administered daily over a six-week period. Traveling long distances can take a toll on you, physically and emotionally.

In many cases, you'll find a facility that meets both criteria. If not, you may decide that having access to the best equipment takes precedence, and that you can figure out a way to handle the travel.

Advances in Radiation Therapy

New techniques are making treatment safer and more effective all the time.

The discovery of radiation and its effect on cancer cells in the late 19th and early 20th centuries created a new and powerful branch of modern medicine. Today, computer-assisted techniques offer hope for people with cancers that were previously considered difficult, if not impossible, to treat with conventional medicine. And advanced radiation therapy techniques make it possible to heal certain cancers, such as some breast and prostate cancers, in less invasive ways.

STATE-OF-THE-ART MEDICINE

Intensity modulated radiation therapy (IMRT) is one of the most important breakthroughs in external radiation. This technique has proven especially effective in the treatment of difficult-to-reach cancers, and those located close to delicate organs. Using a powerful computer program, the oncologist can plan a precise dose of radiation in three dimensions, based on the size, shape, and location of the tumor. IMRT delivers radiation in thousands of thin beams that enter the body from hundreds of angles, intersecting the cancer with great precision.

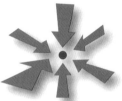

IMRT

A few patients receive **radioactive isotopes** orally as part of their treatment plan. Radioactive isotopes are elements that are unstable, so that they emit radiation.

For example, Iodine-131 is an unstable, or radioactive, form of the element iodine that is used as a post-surgical treatment for thyroid cancer. The thyroid absorbs the Iodine-131, which gives off radiation and destroys the remaining cancer cells.

YOUR RADIATION TEAM

Your radiation team includes a number of highly trained doctors, specialists, and caregivers who work with you throughout your treatment:

The **radiation oncologist** is a doctor who specializes in treating cancer with radiation therapy, and who will determine and oversee your treatment

The **radiation physicist** helps the radiation oncologist design and implement treatment and ensures proper functioning of equipment

Another high-technology approach is **3-D conformal radiation**. Using three-dimensional computer mapping, the oncologist produces an accurate image of the tumor and surrounding organs, so that multiple radiation beams can be shaped exactly to the contour of the tumor. This method can accurately deliver high doses of radiation, and it has been used to treat many cancers, including prostate, lung, and certain brain tumors.

Gamma knife radiosurgery is an advanced form of radiotherapy that's used to treat brain tumors. Also known as **stereotactic surgery**, this procedure uses hundreds of extremely precise beams of radiation to target the brain tumor. Instead of receiving therapy in multiple sessions, however, the gamma knife procedure requires only one high-dose session.

BREAKTHROUGHS IN BRACHYTHERAPY

High dose rate (HDR) brachytherapy is a new innovation in internal radiation. Some cancer facilities are now able to use computers to deliver a few powerful but precise doses of radiation to the site of the tumor over a few short outpatient treatments. The entire treatment takes only a day or two, and poses very little risk of radiation injury to normal tissue. For some cancers, HDR may be just as effective as surgery for treating the entire tumor.

Another recent advance in brachytherapy holds great promise for people with breast cancer. **MammoSite® radiation therapy (MRT)** is used after a **lumpectomy**, or the surgical removal of a breast tumor, and enables doctors to deliver radiation where cancer is most likely to recur. The oncologist inserts a small, balloon-shaped catheter into the cavity where the tissue was removed. Then the oncologist loads the catheter with a tiny radioactive pellet. You can receive treatment as an outpatient, usually over one to five days. MRT is far less invasive than external radiation, and can help doctors preserve as much of the healthy breast tissue as possible.

The **dosimetrist** helps the radiation oncologist formulate treatment and determine techniques such as angle of radiation entry and daily radiation dose

The **radiation therapist** operates the equipment and positions you for treatment

The **radiation therapy nurse** has extensive experience working with people who are undergoing radiation treatment

SIDE EFFECTS

Unlike chemotherapy, radiation is a local treatment, which means side effects are usually limited to the area of the body that's receiving radiotherapy. Almost all side effects are temporary, and thanks to improved techniques, people are finding radiation easier to tolerate. Here are some of the most common:

- **Fatigue.** This is a sign that your body is fighting hard against the cancer. Good nutrition and adequate rest will help your body heal.

❝Thousands of people who have had radiation therapy alone or in combination with other types of cancer treatment are free of cancer.❞
National Cancer Institute

- **Skin irritation.** This is an occasional side effect of external radiation, usually limited to the area where radiation passes through the skin.

- **Nausea and diarrhea.** These can sometimes be a problem for people receiving radiation in the abdominal or pelvic area, and sometimes to the brain.

Discuss side effects with your doctor. There are many medications and natural therapies available that can relieve symptoms.

TO LEARN MORE
Radiation Therapy and You: A Guide to Self-Help During Cancer Treatment
www.cancer.gov/cancerinfo/Radiation-therapy-and-you
National Cancer Institute website

Immunotherapy

Immunotherapy reinforces your body's power to protect itself.

Surgery, chemotherapy, and radiation have long been considered the three most powerful weapons in the fight against cancer. In recent years, **immunotherapy**—also called **biological therapy** or **biological response modifier** therapy—has taken its place alongside other conventional therapies as an effective treatment for some types of cancer. This promising new treatment builds on what scientists understand about the immune system's role in the development and prevention of disease. Cancer can develop when the immune system becomes damaged or compromised and can't defend your body adequately against illness. Biological therapy stimulates the immune system to help it fight cancer more effectively.

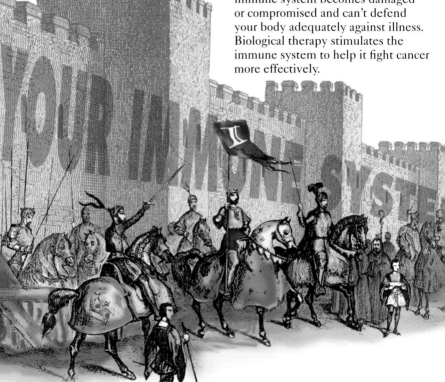

SENDING IN REINFORCEMENTS

Biological therapies can work in a variety of ways. Some of them make the cancer appear more foreign to your body, activating an immune response. Others attack the tumor directly, or stimulate specific cells of your body to attack it. Many improve the overall activity and energy of the immune system, increasing the odds that your body will recognize and destroy cancerous cells.

Immunotherapy is usually administered intravenously. Treatment may last from two weeks to several months, or possibly a year. Here are some of the most widely used therapies:

Monoclonal antibodies are used to treat leukemia, lymphoma, and some solid tumors. Your doctor will analyze your cancerous cells to detect **antigens** on their surface. These antigens are matched with laboratory-made **antibodies** that attach to the antigens and destroy the cancer cells or stop them from reproducing. You may receive the antibodies alone, or as carriers of other therapeutic substances. For instance, chemotherapy agents may be attached to the antibodies, delivering chemo directly to the cancer cells. This technique may help make chemotherapy

> **"** *Many members of the medical community view immunotherapy as the most promising new means of controlling cancer in the future.* **"**
>
> Cancer Research Institute

A SOPHISTICATED DEFENSE

The immune system is the human body's complex defense network. Made up of 20 trillion cells, proteins, and other substances, the immune system is your internal, disease-fighting army that recognizes foreign invaders and launches an elaborate attack against them. Your immune system is on the lookout for viruses, bacteria, and diseases such as cancer. Cancer can be especially difficult for your immune system to detect and destroy because cancer cells are damaged cells created by your own body, not foreign invaders such as germs.

Mounting evidence suggests that people become especially susceptible to cancer when the immune system is not working as well as it should.

The paradox of many conventional treatments, such as chemotherapy and radiation, is that while they destroy tumors, they sometimes also weaken your immune system in the process.

During biological therapy, doctors manipulate the cells of your immune system to invigorate its cancer-fighting abilities, or to help it rebound from some of the debilitating effects of other conventional treatments.

NOT WITHOUT CHALLENGES

Biological therapies are a promising, but still experimental, area of treatment. Every day, biologists gain new insights into the immune system, offering hope for more effective ways of curing and managing cancer in the future.

In the meantime, however, immunotherapy can pose a variety of challenges. Because some of these therapies are considered investigational, patients may have difficulty obtaining insurance coverage for their treatment.

Also, while the side effects of some biological therapies tend to be mild, others can produce severe, and occasionally dangerous, reactions. It's important to discuss the risks of treatment with your doctor. Most commonly, people experience flu-like symptoms—signs that your immune system is actively fighting cancer.

CANCER VACCINES

Researchers are working to develop cancer vaccines. Most vaccines prevent disease by exposing the body to a weak version of a virus, spurring the immune system to fight it. That response produces antibodies, which respond to any actual assault. Using the same principle, scientists believe they can stimulate a patient's immune system to fight existing tumors and prevent recurrence. While cancer vaccines are experimental, the research is promising.

TO LEARN MORE

www.cancerresearch.org
Cancer Research Institute website

---

more effective, while reducing toxic side effects.

 Interleukins are widely used as a therapy for melanoma, lymphoma, and kidney cancer. These hormone-like substances stimulate your white blood cells to fight cancer and promote the growth of cancer-destroying cells.

 Interferons are used to treat some blood cancers, melanoma, and AIDS-related Kaposi's sarcoma. Your body recognizes cancerous cells by special marks on their surfaces. Interferons can help make cancer easier for your immune system to recognize, and they prevent the growth of new cancerous cells. Interferons may also help make other treatments, such as radiation therapy and certain chemotherapies, more effective.

 Hematopoietic growth factors are substances that encourage the growth of new blood cells, which are the basis of your immune system. Your doctor may recommend them after chemotherapy or a stem cell transplant to help stimulate the creation of essential blood cells.

Stem Cell Transplant

Pioneering new methods are changing the landscape of stem cell transplant.

Bone marrow—the spongy tissue inside your bones—is where new blood cells are born. Your blood cells perform a variety of functions that are vital to life, such as ferrying oxygen and

STEM CELLS TO THE RESCUE

In a stem cell transplant:

1 Blood is drawn from the patient or a donor

2 Stem cells are harvested from the blood

3 High-dose chemotherapy eliminates cancer cells

4 Introduction of healthy stem cells into the blood replenishes the immune system

other essential elements to your tissues and removing wastes and toxins from them. Blood cells also make up your immune system. Whenever an invader is detected, the cells of your immune system spring into action, surrounding and destroying your body's internal enemies.

Stem cells are immature cells that are produced by the bone marrow and circulate throughout the bloodstream. Stem cells reproduce quickly and stimulate the growth of new blood cells and immune cells in the bone marrow.

If your bone marrow becomes damaged, it may not be able to produce enough stem cells and healthy blood cells to support your body and fight off infection. This can happen if you develop a disease that originates in the blood or the bone marrow, such as **leukemia**.

CREATING A NEW IMMUNE SYSTEM

These hematologic cancers were difficult to treat until the 1970s when a breakthrough procedure known as a **bone marrow transplant (BMT)** was developed. This treatment relies on high doses of chemotherapy to eliminate cancerous bone marrow, after which

TO LEARN MORE
www.marrow.org
National Marrow Donor Program website

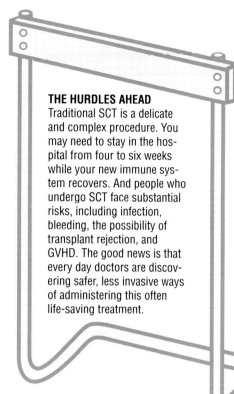

patients receive healthy bone marrow intravenously. This bone marrow contains stem cells that go to work in the patient's body, creating new, healthy bone marrow and blood cells.

In recent years, advanced technology has allowed doctors to remove only stem cells from the bloodstream, transplanting them intravenously to replenish a patient's bone marrow. Most transplants today are **stem cell transplants (SCT)**, although they are still sometimes referred to as bone marrow transplants.

Although the procedure was originally developed to treat people with blood cancers by directly replacing unhealthy bone marrow, today SCT is routinely used to treat solid tumor cancers that are most vulnerable to chemotherapy at very high levels. Since chemotherapy can damage bone marrow at high doses, SCT is used to repair that damage. Transplanted stem cells create a new, healthy immune system. When SCT is used in this manner, it is sometimes called **stem cell rescue**. For people whose cancer might be cured with aggressive conventional therapy, stem cell transplant offers a cause for hope.

A GOOD MATCH
There are two main types of stem cell transplant:

Autologous transplants use your own stem cells, which are removed and stored, and returned to your body after you receive high-dose chemotherapy.

Allogeneic transplants use stem cells from a volunteer donor, usually a member of your immediate family.

The success of an allogeneic transplant often depends on how closely the donor's stem cells match your own. If your body recognizes the cells as foreign, it may reject the transplant, which can result in serious, sometimes life-threatening complications, including organ damage. It's also possible that the transplanted stem cells will recognize your body as foreign, and react against it. This is known as **graft versus host disease**, or GVHD. Siblings are almost always the closest match,

THE HURDLES AHEAD
Traditional SCT is a delicate and complex procedure. You may need to stay in the hospital from four to six weeks while your new immune system recovers. And people who undergo SCT face substantial risks, including infection, bleeding, the possibility of transplant rejection, and GVHD. The good news is that every day doctors are discovering safer, less invasive ways of administering this often life-saving treatment.

and scientists have developed a highly sophisticated process, called **HLA typing**, for matching donors. HLA typing matches your genetic material and the proteins on your cells' surfaces to those of a potential donor.

MINI-TRANSPLANTS
Some facilities are now investigating milder, less toxic approaches to SCT. One promising new method is the **non-myeloablative** transplant, sometimes called the **mini-transplant**.

During a traditional SCT, the patient receives high doses of chemotherapy before treatment to destroy the existing cancerous cells. Mini-transplants use lower and less toxic doses of chemotherapy. While some cancer cells may remain, the newly transplanted cells recognize the cancer cells as foreign and attack them.

Stem cell transplant has a reputation as a treatment of last resort, used only after other conventional therapies have failed. But in fact, SCT may be used to treat people with recurrent but minimal cancer that responds well to aggressive chemotherapy. In addition to blood cancers, SCT may also be used to treat solid tumor cancers, such as breast, ovarian, kidney, and testicular cancer.

Other Advances in Treatment

New treatments zero in on cancer cells' vulnerabilities.

As scientists learn more about cancer, they're developing promising new therapies that target specific types of tumor cells and inhibit their growth. On their own or in combination with other conventional treatments, such as chemotherapy and radiation, these therapies can reduce the size of some tumors and alleviate patients' symptoms. Some new therapies offer hope for people with cancers that have been resistant to more mainstream treatments.

THE MORE WE KNOW

Every day scientists learn more about how certain tumors grow and how to stop them from growing. **Hormone therapy**, for example, emerged from a better understanding of what substances some tumors need to survive: By cutting off the supply of those substances, doctors may be able to stop cancer in its tracks. And the discovery that some tumor cells are vulnerable to heat led to the development of **hyperthermia** and **radiofrequency ablation** therapies.

Chemoembolization

Liver tumors—both primary and **metastatic**—can be notoriously difficult to treat with surgery. Chemo-embolization is a local therapy that can reduce the size of these cancers. By threading a catheter through the main artery that feeds the liver, the onco-logist delivers

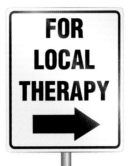

a powerful dose of chemotherapy directly to the organ. Special oils are also fed through the catheter that block the flow of blood to the tumor. This starves it of the nutrients and oxygen it needs to grow, and traps the chemotherapy inside the liver, where it's needed most. While che-moembolization is still considered an investigational therapy, many people have experienced a reduction of symp-toms and, in some cases, an improved prognosis with this treatment.

Hormone Therapy

Certain cancers, including some breast and prostate cancers, need hormones such as estrogen and testosterone to grow. Removing a tumor's supply of these hormones can slow down, and sometimes stop, the reproduction of cancerous cells. For instance, the drug tamoxifen reduces the ability of estro-gen to stimulate hormone-responsive cancers such as breast cancer.

Another form of hormone therapy is to surgically remove the ovaries or the testicles, which are the organs that pro-duce the hormones.

Hormone therapy can cause physical and psychological side effects, includ-ing loss of fertility, a change in sexual desire, or early menopause in women. The side effects you could experience will depend on the type of therapy you're undergoing. Many people find that some side effects disappear as their bodies grow accustomed to treatment. Others find ways, over time, of adapting to physical changes.

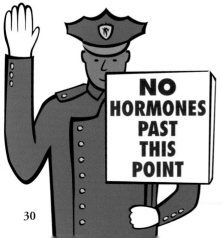

Some targeted therapies are still considered investigational, and may only be available at a few specialized or state-of-the-art cancer facilities. If you're interested in a specific therapy, talk to your oncologist about where you might be able to receive treatment.

Hyperthermia

Hyperthermia treatments raise the temperature of a tumor to 106° or more—high enough to damage its cells. Your doctor may heat the tumor using external applicators or insert wires into the tumor under anesthesia.

Hyperthermia is most effective when it's used in combination with chemtherapy and radiation, since heat makes the cancer cells more sensitive to these therapies. Used to treat a variety of cancers, including those of the skin, prostate, and breast, hyperthermia can sometimes cause blisters or burns.

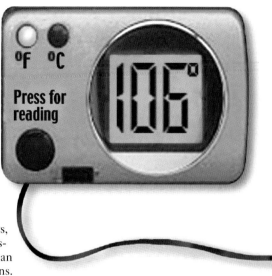

Radiofrequency Ablation

Radiofrequency ablation (RFA) is another treatment that manipulates cancer cells' vulnerability to heat. Designed for treatment of liver cancers that cannot be removed surgically, RFA uses a special catheter to deliver electrical energy—similar to microwaves—directly to the tumor. As the temperature of the tumor cells rises above 113°, their cell structures become damaged, and they die almost immediately. For many people with liver cancer, RFA is a fast, effective, and relatively low-risk alternative to more standard treatments.

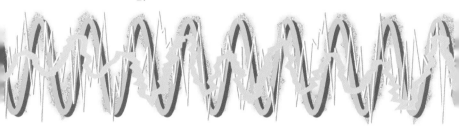

Photodynamic Therapy (PDT)

Scientists have discovered certain non-toxic chemicals that make tumor cells vulnerable to light. These chemicals, called **photosensitizing agents**, are injected into your bloodstream and become concentrated in the cancerous cells. Then your doctor shines a special light onto your tumor, destroying the now light-sensitive cells. **PDT** has been used successfully to treat many types of skin cancer, esophageal cancer, and some lung cancers.

❝ *Potential new solutions to the problem of cancer seem limited only by the imagination. In some promising new therapies, the body's internal weapons are trained on cancerous growths. In other treatments, no less a powerful element than light is employed to eradicate the invaders.* **❞**
National Cancer Institute

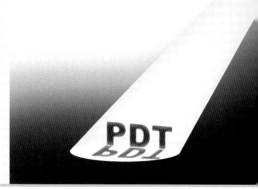

Complementary Therapies

Your choice of cancer treatments isn't limited to what's conventional.

Conventional medicine is the foundation of most people's cancer treatment. However, studies show that more than 70% of people with cancer use some form of non-traditional, or **complementary**, therapy in addition to their primary treatment. For instance, patients turn to therapies as diverse as **acupuncture, homeopathy,** and **aromatherapy** to supplement their medical care.

Certain therapies are especially effective cancer-fighters since they are proven to reinforce the immune system—the first line of defense against cancer—and enhance overall health. **Complementary and alternative medicine (CAM)** approaches, such as **naturopathic medicine, nutritional therapy, physical therapy,** and **mind-body medicine**, are gaining wide acceptance as indispensable aspects of a comprehensive cancer treatment plan.

same treatment may be considered **alternative** if it is used instead of conventional treatment.

NEW PERSPECTIVES
Many CAM therapies are based on concepts of wellness and disease that are profoundly different from those of Western medicine. For instance, **traditional Chinese medicine (TCM)** is a CAM therapy that is used to treat millions of people in Asia. Central to TCM is the concept of *Qi* (pronounced "chee"). *Qi* is usually translated as "life force" or "vital energy." Practitioners of TCM believe illness is caused by obstructions to the flow of this energy. There is no equivalent to this concept in Western medicine, which usually characterizes disease as a

Conventional therapies
- Surgery
- Chemotherapy
- Immunotherapy
- Radiation
- Stem cell transplants

IT'S HOW YOU USE IT
Broadly speaking, CAM is the extremely diverse range of therapies outside of conventional medicine. They were developed all over the world, many from non-Western medical philosophies. Some are thousands of years old, while others are more recent developments.

A therapy may be complementary or alternative depending on how it's used. Therapies are considered **complementary** when they're used in addition to conventional treatment to reinforce the immune system, relieve symptoms, and enhance the effectiveness of conventional therapies. The

hostile invader. In fact, one of the benefits of CAM therapies is that they embrace a variety of perspectives on health and illness that can be employed in versatile ways.

CARING FOR THE WHOLE PERSON
Many CAM therapies promote a **holistic** approach to health. This means that they address a person's overall wellbeing rather than just the physical manifestations of illness. CAM therapies often aim to identify and treat the

root causes of disease—including its physical, emotional, spiritual, and mental dimensions—rather than just eradicate symptoms. In addition, CAM therapies can help patients achieve a sense of inner balance and peace.

It is this emphasis on a better quality of life that helps make CAM therapies so popular among cancer patients. Mental, emotional, and spiritual factors all play a role in your health, but most conventional treatments only address physical concerns. Complementary therapies can also reduce side effects, promote overall wellness, and focus on the comfort of patients, making conventional treatment more bearable. CAM therapies themselves are often pleasant, since they're usually natural, non-toxic, and minimally invasive.

BE DISCRIMINATING

It's important to distinguish between legitimate complementary therapies that will bolster your fight against cancer, and those that won't help and may even harm you. Researching therapies with your oncologist or a qualified naturopathic physician are good ways to find out if a particular therapy might be helpful.

You want to be informed of any dangers a particular therapy might pose.

But there's also a chance that you'll find a treatment that, while it has had no proven effect in a scientific study, makes you feel better. Keep an open mind, but make informed treatment decisions by consulting with a naturopathic physician.

In general, be wary of treatments or practitioners who claim to be able to cure cancer. There is no magic pill that eliminates cancer, so if something sounds too good to be true, it probably is. Responsible complementary therapists will encourage you to use their treatments as enhancements to a carefully planned course of conventional treatment. You should also be cautious when considering therapies that are prohibitively expensive. Some unethical individuals try to take financial advantage of cancer patients with costly but ineffective treatments.

> **❝ Natural forces within us are the true healers of disease. ❞**
> Hippocrates

Complementary therapies

- Naturopathic medicine
- Nutritional therapy
- Physical therapy
- Mind-Body medicine
- Spiritual support

Complementary and conventional therapies go hand in hand

A MATTER OF DEBATE

Most experts agree that using CAM therapies as an alternative to conventional medicine can be a risky approach to treating cancer, and would not be recommended by most healthcare practitioners.

For instance, using acupuncture to relieve post-operative pain or nausea after chemotherapy is a complementary therapy endorsed by the National Institutes of Health. But using acupuncture alone to treat cancer itself might be dangerously ineffective.

TO LEARN MORE

Choices in Healing: Integrating the Best of Conventional and Complementary Approaches to Cancer
by Michael Lerner, 1996

Naturopathic Medicine

The power of nature can help your body heal.

More and more doctors, caregivers, and patients are recognizing the important role that naturopathic medicine, or naturopathy, can play in cancer treatment.

Naturopathic medicine is a comprehensive system of healthcare that dates back more than 100 years, although it has its roots in ancient medicine. Founded by a German-American MD, Dr. Benjamin Lust, naturopathic medicine integrates a wide variety of natural therapies that have been clinically proven to strengthen the immune system, improve overall health, and help prevent illness.

Although naturopathic medicine draws from diverse and seemingly quite different healing traditions, they all share certain principles.

THE HEALING POWER OF NATURE
Naturopathic therapies support and restore the body's inherent ability to heal itself.

LICENSED TO PRACTICE
A doctor of naturopathic medicine, or ND, is someone who has an advanced degree in the study of naturopathic medicine. This degree requires undergraduate premedical training, plus four years of graduate study in medical science and naturopathic philosophy and practice. There are currently five accredited naturopathic colleges in North America that can award the ND degree.

Fourteen US states and four Canadian provinces license NDs as primary care physicians, and they are required to pass a licensing exam to practice legally. In many states, however, the practice of naturopathic medicine is unregulated, and some people may use the ND initials without adequate training.

The website of the American Association of Naturopathic Physicians, a professional organization, offers contact information for all licensing boards as well as a database of licensed NDs practicing in all states.

THE PHYSICIAN AS TEACHER
Naturopathic doctors work closely with their patients to help educate and empower them to take control of their health.

FIRST DO NO HARM
Naturopathic medicine emphasizes healing therapies that are natural and non-invasive.

TREAT THE CAUSE
In addition to treating the symptoms of disease, naturopathic medicine seeks to identify and treat the underlying causes of illness.

TO LEARN MORE
www.naturopathic.org
American Association of Naturopathic Physicians website

THE WHOLE PICTURE

Naturopathic medicine is by definition **holistic**. This means that naturopathic doctors evaluate all aspects of your wellbeing, including your physical, emotional, and spiritual health. At the core of the naturopathic tradition is the belief that nutrition is the cornerstone of good health. Along with a healthy diet and supplementation with vitamins, minerals, and other nutrients, naturopathic physicians may also recommend therapies from the disciplines of **botanical medicine, homeopathy, Eastern medicine,** and **psychology,** among others. Many of these treatments have been proven in clinical studies to boost immune system function.

A COLLABORATIVE APPROACH

Studies show that, when used in conjunction with conventional treatment, these natural therapies can improve the outlook for many cancer patients. Oncologists do their best to identify and eliminate any cancer cells in your body. A naturopathic physician complements an oncologist's work by recommending natural, non-invasive therapies that can improve the effectiveness of conventional treatment, restore your sense of wellbeing, and help you take charge of your health in whatever ways you can.

For example, a naturopathic doctor may prescribe specific nutritional supplements or botanical therapies that enhance the effectiveness of radiation or chemotherapy, while reducing their side effects. And naturopathic doctors work with you to help you make lifestyle or dietary changes that can make you stronger, healthier, and better able to benefit from conventional treatment.

COMPATIBLE VIEWS

While naturopathic medicine is a distinct system of healthcare, that doesn't mean it's opposed to conventional medicine. Cooperation between disciplines is at the heart of the naturopathic philosophy. Naturopathic physicians often collaborate with and refer patients to conventional medical doctors for diagnosis or treatment.

Reputable naturopathic physicians receive rigorous training in conventional medical disciplines, such as anatomy, biochemistry, pathology, and clinical medicine, as well as natural medicine. During your office visit with a naturopathic doctor, you may undergo extensive lab work, assessments, and medical tests, similar to what you experience when you go for a checkup with a conventional doctor.

TREAT THE WHOLE PERSON
Naturopathic therapies address all aspects of your health, including physical, emotional, spiritual, genetic, and environmental factors.

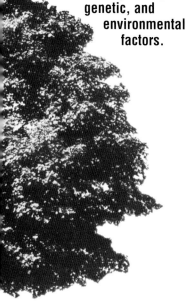

PREVENTIVE MEDICINE
Naturopathic medicine promotes lifestyle habits that strengthen the immune system and prevent illness.

❝ The goal of naturopathic medicine is to retain the best of traditional practice while continuing to evolve as new information becomes available. ❞

American Association of
Naturopathic Physicians

Naturopathic Treatments

A spectrum of therapies support your whole body.

Naturopathic physicians believe that cancer arises from an imbalance that causes a systemic breakdown within the body. NDs help patients restore internal balance and build their resistance to cancer by empowering them to make lifestyle and dietary changes. And NDs prescribe natural therapies that can slow tumor growth, strengthen the immune system, and enhance the effectiveness of conventional therapy.

As with conventional treatment, the naturopathic therapies that are right for you will depend on your diagnosis, your overall state of health, and your primary course of treatment.

GOALS OF NATUROPATHIC MEDICINE

- Provide ongoing, patient-centered healthcare
- Speed recovery from surgery
- Reduce side effects and enhance the effectiveness of chemotherapy and radiation therapy
- Support the immune system
- Maximize the body's absorption of nutrients
- Modulate hormonal levels
- Detoxify the body

A RANGE OF

Naturopathic physicians use a variety of therapies to treat people with cancer, including:

Clinical nutrition. Naturopathic doctors believe that good nutrition is the foundation of good health. Studies show that cancer patients who maintain high-quality nutrition fight off secondary infections, recover more quickly, and tolerate conventional therapy better.

Depending on your needs, your ND will probably recommend dietary changes and may supplement your diet with high-protein shakes and vitamins, minerals, and other nutrients usually taken in pill form.

Botanical medicine. Plants have been used to treat medical conditions since the beginning of civilization. Today, 80% of the world's population uses botanical remedies, and many Western drugs are plant-derived, including some of the most powerful chemotherapy agents.

NDs use plant-based medicines to fortify the body and relieve symptoms. For example, aromatic plants such as **ginger, fennel**, and **mint** can relieve nausea. **Green tea** contains powerful cancer-fighting compounds. Chinese herbs, such as **astragalus**, are often used to relieve symptoms and boost the immune system.

Hydrotherapy. An extremely gentle treatment, hydrotherapy can be used internally to aid elimination of waste products, or externally to stimulate blood flow and boost cellular absorption of nutrients. Many naturopathic physicians recommend that cancer patients drink eight glasses of water a day. Baths and showers at hot and cold temperatures are common forms of external hydrotherapy.

THE BIG EIGHT

In their book, *How to Prevent and Treat Cancer with Natural Medicine*, NDs Michael Murray, Tim Birdsall, Joseph Pizzorno, and Paul Reilly recommend the following natural substances as potent cancer fighters. They should only be taken as part of a comprehensive treatment plan, under the supervision of an ND:

1 **Proteolytic enzymes** are derived from a variety of plant and animal sources. They can slow the spread of cancer in your body, as well as protect against infections.

2 **Curcumin**—the yellow pigment in the spice turmeric—has powerful anti-cancer properties.

3 **Quercetin** is a common flavonoid in many plant foods that helps prevent cancer cells from dividing.

4 **Maitake mushroom extract** stimulates the cells of the immune system.

> ❝ *You'll increase your odds of survival and have a higher quality of life if you take advantage of the whole spectrum of therapies, including those that harness the healing power of nature.* ❞
>
> Michael Murray, ND, Tim Birdsall, ND, Joseph E. Pizzorno, ND, and Paul Reilly, ND, *How to Prevent and Treat Cancer with Natural Medicine*

5 **PSK** and **PSP** are compounds derived from cloud fungus mushrooms that are widely used in Japan and China to treat cancer.

6 **Polyerga** is derived from pig spleens and has been used for over 50 years to treat breast, colon, and other carcinomas.

7 **Modified citrus pectin** is extracted from the peel and pulp of citrus fruits and may help prevent some types of cancer from spreading.

8 **Ip6**, or **Inositol Haxaphosphate**, is a component of fiber that is a powerful anti-oxidant and boosts the immune system.

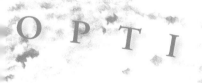

OPTIONS

Homeopathic medicine. Developed in the late 19th century, homeopathy is a system of medicine that uses minuscule doses of plant and mineral substances to treat the symptoms of cancer based on their causes.

Acupuncture and acupressure. Among the best known procedures of traditional Chinese medicine (TCM), acupuncture and acupressure are shown to relieve pain, nausea, and the side effects of hormone therapy for prostate cancer. Both are based on the concept of *Qi*, or the flow of life energy through the body. Acupressure relies on the massage of key energy points within the body to realign *Qi*. Acupuncturists treat patients by painlessly inserting thin needles into strategic points in the body to redirect the flow of energy.

Natural anti-tumor agents. Certain natural substances have been shown to be especially potent in slowing or stopping the growth of tumors. Your naturopathic physician might recommend different agents, or combinations of agents, based on your diagnosis and treatment plan.

STRONG MEDICINE
While most natural medicines are safe, taking certain combinations can produce unwanted side effects or even interfere with treatment. Make sure to discuss any supplements you're considering with your ND and oncologist.

$\mathcal{F}$ood for Living

Wholesome food has healing power.

Studies show that consuming a healthy, varied diet is one of the simplest, yet most powerful, ways to improve your odds against cancer.

A nutritious diet strengthens the immune system, and a healthy immune system can tolerate treatment better and fight cancer more effectively. For instance, some fruits, vegetables, and cold water fish contain nutrients that work in combination with radiation and specific chemotherapy drugs to limit their toxic side effects and enhance their potency.

Many whole, or unprocessed, foods contain nutrients that suppress cancer growth. For instance, brightly colored berries and **cruciferous vegetables**, such as cabbage and broccoli, contain unique agents that can inhibit the development of cancer. In fact, the benefits of consuming adequate amounts of fruit and vegetables are so remarkable that the National Cancer Institute recommends you consume at least five servings a day.

On the other hand, excesses of some foods, such as sugar and **saturated fat**, and inadequate intake of vitamins such as betacarotene, E, C, and folate, may contribute to the development of cancer.

WHEN NUTRITON MAY COUNT MOST

If you have cancer, meeting your nutritional needs may be difficult. That's because cancer releases chemicals into your body that can decrease your appetite while raising your nutritional and caloric requirements. And some types of cancer, as well as many conventional cancer treatments, inhibit your ability to eat, digest food, or absorb nutrients. In addition, many of the side effects of cancer treatment and of cancer itself, such as nausea and fatigue, may further decrease your appetite.

People with cancer who are malnourished experience a reduced

1 Work with a licensed dietitian or nutritionist with oncology experience to design a nutritional plan.

2 Address problems with eating and appetite before they become a health problem. Losing as little as 5% of your body weight is a cause for concern.

3 Even if you're overweight, you may still be at risk for malnutrition because of poor dietary habits. Being overweight may have a negative effect on your recovery. A dietitian can help you design a plan for safe, gradual weight loss.

tolerance to chemotherapy, increased side effects, and a decreased quality of life. Under these circumstances, it's critical to ensure that the food you eat is as nutritionally rich as possible. If you or your caregiver think you're at risk for malnutrition, it's a good idea to talk to a nutritionist.

STEPS TO SUCCESS

Here are four of the key ingredients to a healthy diet:

Eat a variety of whole foods. There is no one miracle food or nutrient that can beat cancer. Your body needs all the essential nutrients, vitamins, minerals, and other elements that can only be found in a varied, natural diet.

Curb your sweet tooth. Processed, sugary foods contain little in the way of nutrients that your body needs. Try snacking on fresh fruits and vegetables instead.

Get adequate lean protein. Whether it comes from fish, soy, legumes, high-protein shakes, or lean poultry and meat, eat a serving of lean protein at every meal.

Trim your fat intake. Diets high in total fat, especially **saturated fat**, are associated with cancer. Opt for healthier sources of fat, such as fish, flaxseed, and olive oils. Avoid **hydrogenated fats**, including margarine, shortening, and refined vegetable oils.

TO LEARN MORE
www.eatright.org
American Dietetic Association website

THE RIGHT STUFF

Some foods are especially rich in the nutrients that support your immune system and have natural cancer-fighting properties:

Green leafy and brightly colored vegetables, including beets, yams, spinach, and tomatoes get their colors from phytochemicals, plant compounds that have potent anti-cancer effects.

Cabbage, cauliflower, and other **cruciferous vegetables** radically lower cancer incidence in laboratory studies.

Cold water fish, such as salmon, sardines, and tuna, provide muscle-building protein, minerals, and omega-3 fatty acids that are beneficial for preventing malnutrition.

Legumes, including soy, garbanzo, black beans, and lentils are high in soluble fiber, which reduces the risk of cancer by helping the body regulate cholesterol and blood sugar levels.

Kelp and other **sea vegetables** contain natural detoxifiers, anti-carcinogens, and essential minerals.

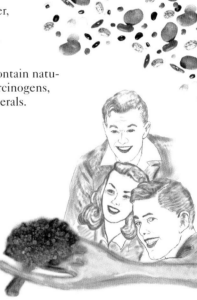

> *"Let food be thy medicine."*
> Hippocrates

Berries, including raspberries, blueberries, and dark cherries contain a powerful anti-cancer agent that causes cancer cells to self-destruct.

Green tea is packed with phytochemicals and other agents that may prevent some cancers.

For patients who can tolerate them, **aromatic foods and spices**, such as garlic, onions, ginger, cayenne, and curry powder add flavor without excess fat and salt, and contain powerful, immune-stimulating compounds.

More than any other food, **dried fruits** like prunes, raisins, and apricots strengthen your blood's ability to protect healthy cells from damage.

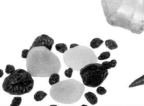

Mind-Body Medicine

Your mind is a powerful force for healing.

Since your diagnosis, you've probably ridden an emotional rollercoaster. It's completely natural to alternate between feeling scared and angry, anxious and hopeful. These are normal emotions, and it's okay to feel and express all of them.

THE MIND-BODY CONNECTION

Cancer doesn't just change your body—having a physical illness affects your thoughts and feelings. **Psychoneuroimmunology (PNI)** is an emerging field of research into the complex interactions of the mind and the immune system. PNI research shows that expressing or releasing your emotions, along the whole spectrum from joy to anger and sadness, can bolster your immune system.

This doesn't mean that being happy—or being angry—will cure your cancer. Nor does it mean that if it's hard for you to express what you're feeling you're making yourself ill. What it does mean is that recognizing and taking care of your emotional needs may help you respond to your physical treatment.

HELPING YOUR MIND, HEALING YOUR BODY

Drawing on PNI research, mind-body medicine aims to strengthen your immune system by helping you deal with the emotional aspects of your illness. Its goals are especially relevant to people with cancer—feeling angry, frustrated, or sad comes with the territory. In addition, people with cancer face all kinds of stressful circumstances, such as resolving finan-

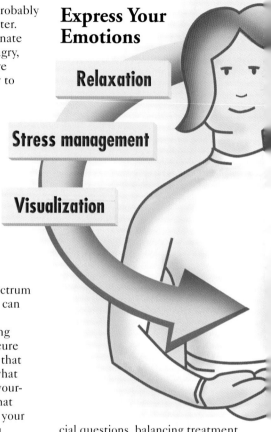

Express Your Emotions

Relaxation

Stress management

Visualization

cial questions, balancing treatment and work, and coping with not feeling well. Sometimes, just realizing it's natural to feel rage or depression about your illness can help you feel better.

Taking good care of yourself is one of the most important things you can do to help yourself during this stressful time. This means treating yourself as you would treat a good friend dealing with cancer. Being hard on yourself can hamper your ability to cope with the illness.

GETTING THE SUPPORT YOU NEED

Talking with professional counselors, other people with cancer, and family and friends can remind you that you're not alone and help you cope with the emotional aspects of your illness.

Support groups are made up of cancer patients and survivors who meet and discuss their common experiences. Research shows that patients who communicate with other people

> **❝** Never forget the importance of being good to yourself as you go through the cancer experience. Doing so will help you deal with your illness most effectively. **❞**
>
> Katherine L. Puckett, LCSW

Seek Support from Others

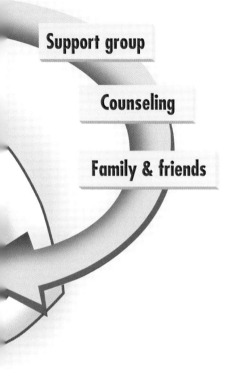

Support group

Counseling

Family & friends

who've had similar experiences are better able to cope with their cancer.

Individual or **group counseling** is provided by a social worker, psychologist, or psychiatrist. The therapist can help you express your feelings and worries and provide emotional coping techniques.

Family and **friends** may be a great source of support and comfort. If those who are closest to you find it difficult to deal with their own feelings or to know how best to support you, it may be very helpful for you to let them know what you need from them.

FINDING FOCUS

Dealing with cancer is one of the most stressful experiences a person can face. There are a variety of techniques you can use to help you relax and focus on feeling better.

Meditation is a spiritual practice that can also be used therapeutically. When you meditate, you focus all of your attention on one thought, helping you release tension. You might find that you prefer to relax and focus your thoughts through prayer, time spent enjoying nature, or practicing yoga or tai chi. All these forms of meditation can help reduce stress and relieve pain.

Visualization and **guided imagery** use relaxation and imagination to focus your mind on healing. During visualization, you may picture your immune system destroying cancer cells or imagine yourself in a peaceful or relaxing place. Some studies suggest that patients who practice visualization feel better and heal faster.

THERE'S NO RIGHT WAY TO COPE

Research shows that releasing emotions strengthens the immune system and increases pain tolerance. For some people, a hearty dose of laughter is a great way to release emotions, and relieve some of the stress of treatment. If you're one of those people, you might feel good after watching your favorite sit-com, renting a funny film, or spending time with a friend who makes you laugh.

Other people, however, find it hard to be light-hearted during cancer treatment, or just don't feel like laughing. It's equally okay not to be upbeat—and it's not bad for your health. You may have to point that out to family or friends, who, with the best intentions, may want you to stay focused on the bright side.

LET IT OUT
Has anyone ever told you that you'd feel better after a good cry? In fact, there is scientific evidence behind the folk wisdom. Releasing your emotions, whether they're feelings of happiness, sadness, or anger, is good for you. When you have a good cry, laugh with pleasure, or express angry feelings, you release **endorphins**, or anti-stress hormones. Endorphins relieve stress and block pain, slow down the effects of aging, and enhance the immune system.

$\mathcal{S}$pirituality

You may find comfort in nurturing your spiritual side.

If you're a spiritual person, you may have long felt a connection between your beliefs and your physical well-being. Now, new research shows spirituality and religion play a vital role in helping people cope with illness, both mentally and physically.

SOURCES OF SPIRITUALITY

When you think about spirituality, you probably associate it with organized religion. For lots of people, belonging to a church, synagogue, mosque, or other religious community connects them to their faith and other people who share their beliefs. Others consider themselves part of a religious community, but express their faith through private prayer.

But organized religion is just one form of spirituality. Many people who don't practice a religion find that certain activities or rituals shift their thoughts from daily worries and connect them to a higher power. For instance, some people find that practicing yoga or meditation, walking in the woods, or listening to beautiful, soothing music may bestow a sense of inner peace even if they don't consider themselves religious. Spirituality is about realizing you're not alone, and that you can turn to some larger force for help, support, or comfort.

Spirituality and religion may become even more important during times of crisis like a serious illness. You've probably wondered at some point since your cancer diagnosis, *Why me?* For some, religion helps to answer that question. Other patients find that prayer helps them make it through the tougher parts of treatment or gives them peace of mind.

While some religions advocate relying on prayer alone as a source of healing, most doctors do not recommend this. Instead, they believe that faith and prayer can be effective complements to modern medicine. Most religious leaders would agree that it is important to seek both medical and spiritual care for your cancer.

SPIRITUALITY AND HEALING

Scientific studies show that religion and spirituality can have a positive influence on health. People who pray or participate in other spiritual practices may tolerate treatment better and experience fewer side effects.

While it's hard to know exactly why this is true, many experts suggest that spiritual practice provides a support system—a social group, a community that shares the same values, and a life philosophy—that imparts a sense of wellbeing and belonging. Studies show that the practice of prayer can actually have a positive effect on a variety of physical processes, including healing and recovery time and the reproduction rate of cancer cells.

These benefits aren't necessarily restricted to the religious setting, however. Studies suggest that people who practice meditation therapeutically may live longer and enjoy improved health. Other relaxation techniques can help alleviate stress, anxiety, and pain. How you choose to express your spirituality is highly personal.

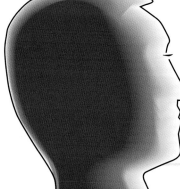

A sense of spirituality can help you realize you're not alone, and that you can turn to a larger force for help, support, or comfort.

FINDING YOUR OWN SPIRITUALITY

There are many different ways you can express your spirituality and enjoy its health benefits:

Attend your church, temple, or mosque. 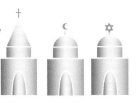 Taking part in an organized religious community can give you practical, moral, and spiritual support. Shared religious practices can also bring families and friends closer together during times of crisis. Participating in prayer may support your healing.

Pray or meditate on your own. Besides being relaxing, prayer and meditation provide positive ways to cope with negative feelings and fears and may give you a sense of peace.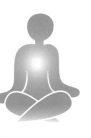

Get in touch with nature. Something as simple as taking a walk in a pleasant park or in the countryside can help you connect with the beauty of the natural world, and give you a sense of calm and peace. Some see nature as a reminder of their place in the universe or as the promise of regeneration.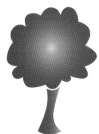

Look to art, music, and writing. Paint a picture, play the piano, or write down your feelings in a journal. Anything that helps you express your emotions may make you feel better. Listening 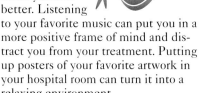 to your favorite music can put you in a more positive frame of mind and distract you from your treatment. Putting up posters of your favorite artwork in your hospital room can turn it into a relaxing environment.

Spiritual counseling. If you already have a relationship with a member of the clergy, he or she can play a comforting, supportive role during your illness. 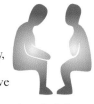 Additionally, most hospitals have a pastor or chaplain on staff. Even if you're not a member of the same faith, religious counselors can be comforting to talk to, and they have lots of experience helping cancer patients cope.

> **"**Whether you choose to express your faith through church attendance, prayer, meditation, or by observing nature, spirituality can be a sound way to cope with your cancer treatment and recovery. **"**
>
> Kim Dalzell, PhD, RD, LD
> *Challenge Cancer and Win!*

TO LEARN MORE
www.nihr.org
International Center for the Integration of Health and Spirituality website

Caring for Your Body

Exercise gives your immune system a boost.

When you're not feeling well, exercise is probably the last thing on your mind. But supporting the body through gentle or moderate exercise and physical activity offers countless benefits for cancer patients. A strengthened body tolerates treatments better and heals faster. Plus, patients who find ways to stay active tend to feel calmer and more confident. Once you're finished with treatment, regaining physical strength is a speedy way back to your normal life.

AN OUNCE OF PREVENTION
Numerous studies show that exercise lowers the risk of cancer and cancer recurrence. For instance, some research suggests that women who work out are less likely to develop breast cancer. Exercise can even reduce the danger for people who smoke or are at high risk for cancer for other reasons.

One reason that active people are less likely to develop cancer is that exercising strengthens the immune system, which is the body's natural defense against disease. Even moderate exercise improves immune function, helping you to fight off infection and other illnesses.

ENHANCING YOUR TREATMENT
Exercise also benefits people who have been diagnosed with cancer:

1. An immune system strengthened by exercise improves response to conventional treatments like chemotherapy and radiation.

2. Moderate physical exercise increases blood flow to the muscles, lessening fatigue and boosting your energy level.

3. Studies show that cancer patients who participate in exercise have a better quality of life. Exercise helps reduce pain and nausea while increasing endurance and improving mood.

4. Physical activity promotes the production of red blood cells and can increase endorphin levels.

While it may seem difficult to find the motivation and energy to exercise

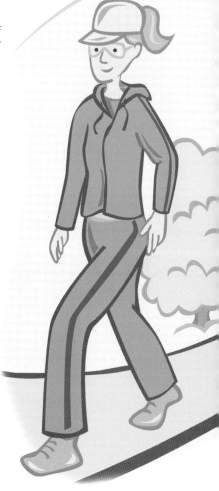

during cancer treatment, something as simple as going for a walk may help you feel better. Even if you're only able to walk for ten minutes at a time, don't give up—any effort you make will be beneficial. And as you continue your routine, you may find that your strength and stamina increase.

> **❝** *Exercise is never more important than when trying to help your body recover from cancer.* **❞**
>
> Michael T. Murray, ND,
> Tim Birdsall, ND, Joseph E.
> Pizzorno, ND, and Paul Reilly, ND,
> *How to Prevent and Treat Cancer
> with Natural Medicine*

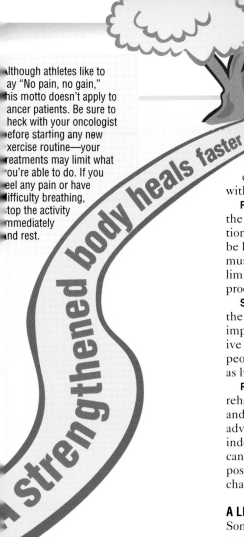

A strengthened body heals faster

Although athletes like to say "No pain, no gain," this motto doesn't apply to cancer patients. Be sure to check with your oncologist before starting any new exercise routine—your treatments may limit what you're able to do. If you feel any pain or have difficulty breathing, stop the activity immediately and rest.

GETTING BACK TO YOUR LIFE

It's also essential to take care of your body once you've finished your cancer treatment. Exercise rebuilds muscle tissue and keeps your immune system at peak function, which can help prevent a recurrence. Moving your limbs regularly will combat any joint stiffness that might be a result of bed rest after surgery, for instance.

For some patients, a healthcare professional like a physical therapist will guide them through the process of physical rehabilitation.

Rehabilitation can be:

Preventive. The goal of preventive rehabilitation is anticipating and limiting impairments that may arise from treatment or a chronic health condition. Patients isolated for prolonged

TO LEARN MORE
The Force Program: The Proven Way to Fight Cancer Through Physical Activity
   by Jeff Berman, Fran Fleegler, MD, and John Hanc, 2001

periods because of a stem cell transplant, for example, may become deconditioned. This can be minimized with an appropriate exercise program.

Restorative. Aiming to re-establish the patient's previous level of function, restorative rehabilitation may be helpful for patients who develop muscle weakness, **lymphedema**, and limited motion following a surgical procedure such as a mastectomy.

Supportive. Along with maximizing the abilities of patients with new impairments or disabilities, supportive rehabilitation also helps educate people about long-term concerns such as lymphedema.

Palliative. The goal of palliative rehabilitation is to provide comfort and support and to help patients with advanced disease be more physically independent. For example, if patients can move from a sitting to a standing position on their own, there's a better chance that home care is viable.

A LITTLE MEANS A LOT

Some people—for example, those who are confined to bed—find that even moderate activity is a challenge. For people with limited mobility, a physical therapist can recommend simple, gentle exercises that can be performed in a chair, or even in bed.

Strengthening. Resistive bands are lengths of stretchy rubber that provide resistance to help build muscle strength and tone. They are one form of exercise that's accessible to many patients.

Aerobic. Walking, swimming, climbing stairs, and cycling are examples of aerobic activity that can help build endurance and decrease fatigue.

Stretching. Simple stretching exercises can be done as a warm up to prepare the body for exercise and to cool down afterwards.

A SOOTHING TOUCH

Massage therapy, or the gentle kneading and manipulation of the muscles, has physical and psychological benefits for some cancer patients. Studies show that massage can reduce pain and anxiety, and instill a sense of well-being, peace of mind, and comfort.

Pain Management

Conquer pain and improve the quality of your life.

Pain is one of the things people with cancer fear most. In fact, for the majority of patients, pain doesn't have to go hand in hand with cancer. Many people with early stage tumors feel little, if any, pain. And according to the American Cancer Society, 90% of people who experience cancer pain are able to find relief.

In the past, however, the majority of cancer pain went unreported and untreated. To combat this situation, many cancer organizations began to raise awareness about how to manage pain effectively. Now, many large hospitals and specialized cancer facilities have pain clinics devoted exclusively to helping patients feel better. Even if yours doesn't, your doctors should suggest a number of alternatives to help you manage any pain you might experience. If your doctor isn't addressing your discomfort, ask to be referred to a pain specialist.

THE ADDICTION MYTH

Many patients avoid pain medication out of fear of addiction. But addiction to painkillers is extremely rare among cancer patients, and people with chronic pain can safely remain on medication for years. Don't let fear of addiction stop you from seeking the relief you need. If you have a history of addiction problems, talk to a pain specialist. He or she can help you find relief.

UNDERSTANDING PAIN

In medical terms, pain is any experience that is unpleasant to the mind and senses. Pain can be **acute** or **chronic**. Acute pain is brief and sharp, while chronic pain lasts longer and may feel duller. Cancer patients might feel both acute and chronic pain at different times—and both are treatable.

Cancer-related pain is often caused by the tumor itself, which may be pressing on nerves or organs. Pain can also be a side effect of some conventional treatments. It's important to keep in mind that increased pain is not necessarily a sign that your cancer is getting worse.

If you notice any pain, you should discuss it immediately with your doctors and nurses. Don't worry about being a complainer or wasting the doctor's time. Your quality of life is important, and there is no benefit to suffering stoically. In fact, patients whose pain goes untreated are less likely to complete their therapy.

For some patients, symptoms like agitation, anger, and stress can actually be signs of untreated pain. Even if your discomfort doesn't seem to be physical, it's worth consulting a pain specialist about ways to control it.

NATURAL RELIEF

Many complementary therapies can help alleviate pain. Because muscular tension and stress can intensify pain, achieving a state of deep relaxation through meditation, visualization, or prayer can bring comfort and a sense of wellbeing. Acupuncture, massage, and other therapies stimulate the release of **endorphins**, which are the body's own painkillers.

While natural therapies may not be enough to eliminate all pain, for most patients they reduce the need for analgesics.

Acupuncture. According to studies endorsed by the National Institutes of Health, acupuncture relieves pain

HOW YOUR DOCTOR CAN HELP

You and your doctor will work together to determine the cause of your pain and find the right treatment. It's a good idea to keep a journal, noting when you feel pain, how bad it is, and how long it lasts. Keep track of any activities that worsen the pain, as well as those that help you feel better.

1 Conventional treatment. Chemotherapy, radiation, and surgery can shrink or eliminate a tumor, relieving pain caused directly by cancer.

2 Medications. Drugs known as analgesics alleviate pain for nearly 90% of cancer patients. These range from mild drugs like aspirin to stronger prescriptions like morphine.

While analgesics can be effective ways of managing pain, patients may initially feel drowsy or in a mental fog. If this continues more than two or three days, and you have

TO LEARN MORE
www.painfoundation.org
American Pain Foundation website

trouble functioning because of your pain medication, talk to your doctor about lowering your dose and controlling pain through other means, such as complementary therapies.

3 Nerve surgery. A surgeon can inject pain medicine into a nerve to block pain, or cut pain nerves in a particular area of the body.

> **"** *Cancer care is not complete until pain is under control.* **"**
> American Cancer Society

after surgery and nausea associated with chemotherapy.

Distraction. Focusing your mind away from pain—on a friend, a book, or a favorite movie—can help you feel more comfortable.

Hypnosis and self-hypnosis, meditation, and visualization. A calm, focused mind can help you manage pain naturally. Talk to a social worker or mind-body therapist to learn self-hypnosis techniques, which have been proven effective at alleviating discomfort.

Massage, heat, and cold therapy. Stimulating the skin with massage, heating pads, or ice packs can provide relief.

Prayer. Prayer counters stress and promotes peace of mind. In fact, for some patients, prayer or meditation may relieve side effects like pain.

Transcutaneous electrical nerve stimulation (TENS). People suffering from acute pain may benefit from TENS, which sends electrical impulses to the affected part of the body.

Music has been advocated as a medical therapy for thousands of years. The ancient Egyptians used music to lessen pain during childbirth. Today's research supports music therapy. One study showed that patients who listened to soothing music after surgery experienced significantly less pain.

47

Comparing Treatment Facilities

Find the finest care for the kind of cancer you have.

Whether you're investigating treatment facilities because you've just been diagnosed with cancer, you're seeking a second opinion, or you're dissatisfied with the place where you're currently being treated, you owe it to yourself to find out where you can get the finest care available for the type of cancer you have.

Oncology programs and the facilities where they're located vary in size, quality, and area of expertise. Among the most significant differences are their technology—specifically whether it is state-of-the-art—and their treatment philosophy. For example, some programs emphasize the integration of nutrition, mind-body medicine, and other types of complementary care. Others do not.

What may complicate your decision is the fact that most oncologists are affiliated with specific hospitals or clinics. So part of choosing an oncologist is considering the facility where you'll be treated.

However, since much of your ongoing treatment may be handled in an outpatient clinic, you may end up working with more than one oncology team and more than one facility— perhaps one in another city and one closer to home.

MAKING A CHOICE

There are excellent cancer facilities of all shapes and sizes. As a general rule, larger hospitals treat more individual cases of cancer each year. Both large and small specialized institutions have pioneered new treatments or approaches and have distinguished reputations. Here's an overview:

University medical centers are teaching hospitals associated with university medical schools. Individual centers may focus on cancer research and treatment. Some well-known cancer specialists are affiliated with particular institutions.

A PATIENT'S CHECKLIST

When you're choosing a treatment facility, here are some of the things to look for:

- Documented experience treating your type of cancer
- Doctors and other caregivers who collaborate across disciplines
- State-of-the-art technology and lab facilities
- Pain management specialists
- Patient services, such as social workers and support groups
- A multi-faceted approach to treatment, including complementary therapies
- Reputable accreditation
- A relationship with a doctor you respect and trust
- A financial partnership with your health insurance provider

Although all hospitals are able to treat pain with drugs and other medical therapies, some have dedicated pain management clinics or specialists. You might want to find out whether the facility you're considering goes the extra mile in helping patients find relief from discomfort.

Keep in mind, though, that some university centers have stronger reputations than others, and that some patients find large hospitals bureaucratic and impersonal.

Community and regional hospitals are extremely diverse. The quality of care varies widely, from excellent to inadequate. If you're diagnosed with a type of cancer that typically responds well to a standard treatment, such a facility may be appropriate. Certain local hospitals are affiliated with university centers and their well-regarded oncologists. Some—but not all—have proper accreditation.

Cancer centers may offer state-of-the-art technology, an experienced staff, and a full range of services, including complementary therapies. Check into the reputation and accreditation of any you're considering. While some are excellent, others may compromise on facilities and staff to keep costs down.

Outpatient clinics may be independent oncology practices or departments of a hospital or cancer center. Most chemotherapy treatments are administered in an outpatient setting, as is most radiation therapy.

A DIFFERENT FOCUS

For some people, a hospital setting may not be the best option.

Home care is an alternative for patients whose illness or living situation makes it difficult for them to get to a hospital. Insurers may reimburse part of the cost for people who are eligible to receive physical therapy and other treatments at home.

Some people with advanced cancer prefer to focus on quality of life rather than continuing with conventional treatment. **Hospice care** manages the symptoms of disease so that people in the late stages of illness can live in comfort and dignity. Hospice care may be given at home, in a hospital, or in a private **hospice center**. When choosing a hospice facility, the most important considerations may be proximity to family and friends, a compassionate staff, and a comforting environment.

SETTING THE STANDARD

Several reputable organizations supervise the quality of cancer care at their member facilities, and some accredit treatment programs:

The National Cancer Institute subsidizes a small number of research hospitals that advance the science of treatment. While NCI cancer centers are not the only place for first-class care, a visit to the NCI website (www.cancer.gov) can be a good starting point for your research.

The American College of Surgeons accredits cancer diagnosis and treatment programs, including research centers, community hospitals, and private clinics. More than 1,450 facilities nationwide meet its stringent standards. You can find out which ones by checking www.facs.org.

The Joint Commission on Accreditation of Healthcare Organizations (JCAHO) reviews most hospitals across the country and accredits them based on staffing, facilities, and safety. Approximately 75% of US hospitals earn JCAHO accreditation, and there's a directory on their website, www.jcaho.org. If the hospital you're considering isn't accredited, find out why.

The Association of Community Cancer Centers (ACCC) is an organization that encourages its member facilities to offer multidisciplinary, state-of-the-art cancer care. The ACCC website (www.accc-cancer.org) provides detailed profiles of its 500 member centers.

A **public hospital** is owned by a local, state, or federal government and is supported by taxes and the fees it charges for its services. A **private hospital**, which may be owned by an institution, such as a university, or by a corporation, is supported by the fees it charges and by grants from the government and other sources.

Working with Your Doctors

Assemble a winning team of cancer experts.

You've probably been visiting doctors since you were a baby. Perhaps you have consulted the same primary care physician (PCP) for most of your adult life. As a cancer patient, you'll have new questions to ask your doctors and new decisions to make about your care.

You're likely to feel more dependent than ever on the professional experience and skill of your doctors. At the same time, you'll want to be sure that you are working with the right team for the type of cancer you have. You may want to ask your PCP why you're being referred to a particular oncologist, or cancer specialist, rather than another. You may have a similar question about whether a local cancer care facility is the best choice for you. You need this information, along with your own research, to make an informed decision.

Your Caregiving Team

It's easy to be confused and sometimes overwhelmed by the number and variety of doctors who are involved in your care. Some cancer patients compare it to the way you feel when you walk into a party where everyone knows each other except you.

The lead doctor in your cancer treatment is often a **medical oncologist**, or doctor who treats cancer using chemotherapy, hormonal therapies, and other medications. Since cancer is a complicated disease, oncologists with different specialties are likely to be part of your healthcare team:

Surgical oncologists focus on using surgery to remove tumors.

Radiation oncologists treat cancer with radiation.

> **"***A good relationship with your doctor is worth the effort it takes to create it.***"**
> American Cancer Society

Gynecological oncologists treat cancers of the female reproductive system.

Immunologists are oncologists who specialize in treating cancer with medications that stimulate and reinforce the immune system.

Often, though not always, these specialists are colleagues and practice in the same hospital or clinic.

My Medical Records

If your oncologist isn't part of a practice that includes your other specialists, you may end up seeing several doctors in different offices over the course of your diagnosis and treatment. Having to wait for each doctor to receive a copy of your medical records before a consultation can delay the momentum and create frustration.

Ask your doctors and nurses for copies of your chart and all of your test results, and take the file with you to each of your appointments. Keeping track of your medical records makes it easier to see other doctors for additional opinions, and it puts you in charge of your own care.

Building a Relationship

It's important to develop a comfortable relationship with your doctors, oncology nurses, and other specialists. It takes time and effort on both ends—just as building any relationship does—and must be built on a foundation of mutual respect.

There are many things you can do to strengthen the relationship:

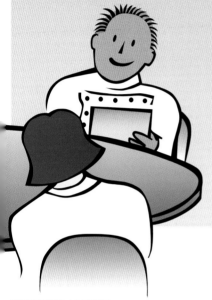

- Be open and straightforward when talking with your doctors and nurses.

- Describe your symptoms thoroughly, using your own words.

- Be honest about your lifestyle, diet, and habits. For example, if you smoke, let them know. Without complete information they can't treat you effectively.

- Let your oncologist know how much information you prefer. You may want all the statistics and results of all the current studies. Or you may want to hear only as much as you need to make informed decisions. But if you don't say which it is, there's no way for your doctor to know.

- You'll also want to know which complementary care providers your doctor works with and how close their collaboration typically is. Explain that you know how important nutrition, naturopathic medicine, mind-body medicine, and other therapies are in the treatment process.

SHOPPING AROUND

Because oncologists are experts, they may be inclined to recommend their own area of expertise as the best way to treat cancer. But it's important to get a second opinion or series of opinions rather than depend solely on one doctor's recommendation. It should not harm your relationship with your primary oncologist if you want another point of view. Most doctors appreciate patients who take a proactive stance toward their healthcare. If you find that's not the case, you may decide you prefer to work with someone different.

It's also worth switching oncologists if you don't seem to click. People have different personalities and communication styles. Maybe your doctor doesn't provide the

encouragement you're seeking, for example, or perhaps his or her treatment philosophy is to watch and wait while you'd rather take action, or the other way around. There's nothing wrong with seeking a more compatible bond.

QUESTIONS FOR YOUR ONCOLOGIST

- What are the goals, benefits, risks, and possible side effects of this treatment?
- How long will the treatment last and what are the chances of a recurrence?
- Why are you recommending this particular treatment for me?
- What are my options if I decide against this treatment?
- Are there any natural therapies that can help me tolerate this treatment?
- How does nutrition affect the way I'll respond to treatment?
- What type of physical activity should I be doing?
- What should I do to prepare myself psychologically and emotionally for treatment?

TO LEARN MORE
Choices
by Marion Morra and Eve Potts, 1994

Paying for Treatment

Persistence and good planning can surmount financial challenges.

If you or a loved one has cancer, confronting the financial cost may seem as overwhelming as fighting the physical and emotional battles. While managing the financial aspects of the illness can be a challenge, it shouldn't deter you from seeking the best care available.

WHAT'S YOUR PLAN?

You may have group health insurance through an employer, association, or professional organization, or you may have an individual policy. In those cases, many of your initial medical expenses may be covered by your plan—provided that the facility you've chosen accepts your coverage. The human resources department at your job and the patient services office at the facility can be great resources at this stage of the process.

You can contact the hospital or clinic directly to find out if they accept your insurance plan. You can also check with the American Cancer Society for a list of facilities that specialize in treating your type of cancer, so you can follow up on which ones accept your plan.

You should also check with your insurer about the limitations the company may impose on your freedom to choose a facility or the additional out-of-pocket costs that may result from choosing one hospital or doctor over another.

☑ Will my insurance cover me at the facility I choose?

☑ What will I have to pay for out-of-pocket?

> **"** No one should ever automatically assume that first-rate care is not available just because money is a problem. **"**
> Cancer Research Institute

MOVING ON

You may want to investigate the type of coverage you may now want or need, especially if you're insured through your job. Many employers offer more than one plan, so you may be able to switch to a more comprehensive alternative at the next enrollment period. If you're married, and your spouse has insurance through his or her employer, you can check to see if that plan is more flexible.

If your medical treatment coverage does not meet your needs, you or your spouse may consider switching jobs if you can find one with better insurance. If you're covered under one employer's plan, the law says you and your dependents are eligible for coverage under a new employer's plan even with a previously existing health problem, as long as employment terms are met.

If your illness means you must leave your job, you can usually continue coverage through the same insurer, under COBRA. However, you must pay the total premium plus an administrative fee.

If you have an individual policy, you may have fewer alternatives if you want to change your policy. New plans can charge higher rates and impose waiting periods before they'll cover your illness.

OLD PLAN

New Plan

BACKUP ARRANGEMENTS

If you don't qualify for, or can't afford, commercial insurance, you may be eligible for public health insurance. Go to your local social services agency or other community organization for help:

Medicare. This federally subsidized program covers people 65 or older or those who have been permanently disabled. Because **metastatic** cancer qualifies as a permanent disability, you may be eligible, although there is a two-year qualifying period. Not all medical providers accept Medicare, so check with your oncologist or facility.

Medicaid. If you're younger than 65, you may qualify for subsidized healthcare through Medicaid, a state-run program for low-income families. You are likely to be limited in your choice of doctors, facilities, and types of treatment. But you will be able to obtain care from Medicare healthcare providers.

Veterans Administration. The Military Health Services System provides medical coverage for veterans who served on active duty, and sometimes their families, in their own facilities. You can contact your local VA office to find out if you're eligible.

TO LEARN MORE
To file a complaint against your insurer, visit the National Association of Insurance Commissioners website: *www.naic.org*

The Patient Advocate Foundation can help you resolve disputes with insurers: *www.patientadvocate.org*

THE FINE PRINT

Most insurance companies refuse to cover therapies they consider experimental or investigational, such as immuno-therapy and stem cell transplant for some cancers.

If an investigational therapy is your best treatment choice, talk to your doctor or hospital social worker about serving as your advocate and helping you appeal your claim:

1. Ask your doctor to send the insurer the research that shows how promising the new treatment is.

2. See if the pharmaceutical company that developed the treatment will lobby on your behalf.

3. Find out if the treatment is part of a clinical trial. If so, some of your costs may be covered.

4. If your appeal is turned down, try to negotiate a lower out-of-pocket cost with your facility.

NEVER GIVE UP
If you feel that you've been unjustly turned down for a claim, you should always appeal.

Keep records. Make copies of all of your insurance claims. Keep your original insurance policy and any addendums. Keep a log of all phone conversations and correspondence with your doctors and insurers. Never submit original documents.

Don't give up. Follow up with your insurer. Double-check your paperwork and re-apply. Many claims are denied because of missing or incorrect documenta-tion, or because a clerk doesn't recognize a code your provider has used. In many cases, the insurer may not request the missing information unless you ask about the status of your claim.

Appeal to your state insurance commissioner. Each state has an office dedicated to monitoring the insurance industry and resolving disputes. Insurers with a pattern of denying claims may be prosecuted.

Your Rights as a Patient

Know your rights, and stand up for them.

You have legal rights as a patient that protect your privacy and access to your medical records. You have rights that protect you against job discrimination because of your illness. Further, you have the right to expect respectful and considerate treatment from your doctors, nurses, and other healthcare providers.

If you feel your rights are being abused but are uncomfortable confronting the issue or afraid it might make your situation worse, enlist the help of a friend or family member who will be more assertive in demanding that the problem is corrected.

Patient's Bill of Rights

In 1973, the American Hospital Association (AHA) drafted a bill of rights for patients, outlining what people being treated for all illnesses should expect to receive from their hospitals, doctors, and nurses. The AHA encourages hospitals and healthcare organizations across the country to comply with the bill of rights, and in many states patients' rights are legally binding.

According to the Patient's Bill of Rights, you are entitled to:

§ **Receive care that is respectful and considerate.**

§ **Be given complete, accurate information in straight-forward language about your diagnosis, prognosis, and treatment plan.**

§ **Make decisions about your treatment, and refuse treatment.**

§ **Expect privacy and confidentiality about your diagnosis and treatment.**

§ **Review and keep a copy of your medical records, and have them explained to you.**

§ **Have access to resources for resolving grievances, disputes, and conflicts.**

§ **Be informed of and understand your rights as a patient at the facility.**

" *Open and honest communication, respect for personal and professional values, and sensitivity to differences are integral to optimal patient care.* **"**

American Hospital Association

EXPECT THE BEST

If you're choosing among treatment facilities, make sure to investigate how well their reputations for patient relationships and their official policies measure up against your treatment philosophy and priorities, as well as the Patient's Bill of Rights.

Most hospitals provide a version of their policies in straightforward language. Federal law requires that any hospital accept- 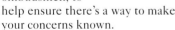 ing Medicare funding inform patients about their legal rights.

But medical facilities should go even further to protect your interests and make you feel comfortable. How they answer your questions and the attitude of the staff as a whole can often tell you a lot about how you'll be treated as a patient.

Some facilities provide patient advocates, or ombudsmen, to 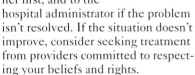 help ensure there's a way to make your concerns known.

If you feel as though your doctor isn't giving you complete information about your diagnosis, for example, or is brushing aside your wishes regarding treatment, you should express your objections to him or her first, and to the hospital administrator if the problem isn't resolved. If the situation doesn't improve, consider seeking treatment from providers committed to respecting your beliefs and rights.

TO LEARN MORE
To see the complete Patient's Bill of Rights, visit the American Cancer Society website:
www.cancer.org

YOUR RIGHTS AS AN EMPLOYEE

When you're worrying about your health, you don't want to worry about your career. Some cancer patients may find their job security threatened as a result of their illness. Others may notice a change in the attitudes of their employers and coworkers, who might be afraid of cancer, or misinformed about how the disease is spread. Although the law can't regulate personal relationships with your coworkers, it does say that you're entitled to fair, professional treatment at your workplace.

For some cancer patients, a lot of job-related anxiety stems from juggling medical appointments, treatment-related fatigue, and a work schedule. Although it can be tricky to find a balance, the law protects you during this stressful time. Your employer is legally required to accommodate your needs while you're being treated for cancer, which can include shifting schedules and assignments and allowing you to work from home.

If you work for a private company of 15 or more employees, you're protected under the Americans with Disabilities Act (ADA). You're also covered by the ADA if you work for a state or local government, employment agency, or labor union. Your employer can't fire you, provide unequal pay or benefits, or otherwise penalize you or treat you differently if you're a qualified cancer patient or cancer survivor.

And if you're looking for a new job, or applying for a job training program, you're entitled to equal consideration with other candidates.

If you feel that you've suffered job discrimination because of your status as a cancer patient or survivor, you can file a complaint with the US Equal Employment Opportunity Commission, or the EEOC, at www.eeoc.gov. You could also contact the Patient Advocate Foundation, at www.patientadvocate. org, for help finding legal representation for employment disputes or financial difficulties.

Your Support Team

Enlist the people you love in your fight against cancer.

There's no time when the love and support of the people you care about is more important than when you have cancer. The team that stands with you—family, friends you've known a long time, or those you've met more recently—wants what's best for you. You can depend on them for emotional support and at times for help with your day-to-day responsibilities. They will also understand that there are things you prefer to handle on your own—if you let them know.

TALKING ABOUT IT

Although it might seem hard at first, being open about your cancer with those you're closest to can alleviate a lot of anxiety for both you and your loved ones. Many people find it helps to share the difficult experience of cancer with close friends and family. Additionally your loved ones probably want to be involved in your daily life, supporting you in any way they can.

You might consider, as you decide whom to tell and when to tell them, if you'll ultimately make the conversation about your health harder if you postpone sharing your diagnosis. At the same time, you should recognize that telling people about your cancer may produce stress of its own. It is an emotional subject, and people don't always know how to react to news that you're ill.

Still, you might be surprised by the amount of comfort and support you find when you begin talking to friends and acquaintances about your experiences. Most people have been close to someone with cancer or another serious illness, and helpful conversations can come from unexpected places.

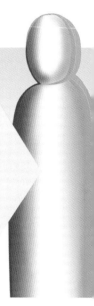

PATIENT

- Being open about your illness can alleviate anxiety

- Turn to supportive family and friends for help and comfort

- Try to be reassuring with kids

- Letting your teenagers help out will give them a sense of control

> **❝** *Family and friends are a very powerful thing. Don't ever underestimate it. We are living proof that a family who shares everything—the good, the bad, and the ugly—can overcome anything, including cancer.* **❞**
>
> Alan Tipple, husband of cancer survivor

ACCEPTING HELP

You may also be more dependent on your family or friends than you've been in the past. Asking for—and accepting—help takes some of the burden off your shoulders and gives them a way to express their love and encouragement. This type of sharing can make relationships even closer.

If people offer to help, don't hesitate to accept. Be specific about the types of things they can do that will make your life easier. They'll be happier knowing they've made a real difference.

TO LEARN MOVE
Taking Time: Support for People with Cancer and the People Who Care About Them
www.cancer.gov/cancerinfo/takingtime
National Cancer Institute website

FAMILY RELATIONSHIPS

Your relationship with your family may grow closer in response to your illness. Or, you might find that your relationships are tense or strained at times even if that wasn't the case before. As husbands, wives, parents, and children take on new responsibilities, they may act differently or step on each others' toes. So it may take a real effort on everyone's part to ease each other's anxieties. Here are some things to try:

- Encourage each other to express frustrations, fears, and even anger.
- Continue the recreational and social activities you've always done together.
- Hold regular family meetings so that everyone can discuss how things are going.
- Consider family counseling to relieve tension or stress.

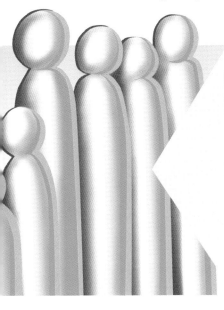

FAMILY & FRIENDS

- Regular family meetings help everyone stay in touch
- Maintaining as normal a routine as possible will put kids at ease
- Spend enjoyable, relaxing time together, such as watching a movie, going for a walk, or just chatting
- Listening, and offering to help, may be what's needed most

SURPRISING REACTIONS

Just as many people will surprise you with their generosity and willingness to help, there's also a chance that a few may surprise you by vanishing from your life. Some people are emotionally unable to cope with a friend's illness and withdraw. Others, suddenly faced with their own vulnerability, may find it easier to avoid you than come to terms with reality. While no one likes to lose touch with friends, it's helpful to acknowledge the loss and move closer to your supporters.

TALKING TO KIDS

If you have young children, it's difficult to tell them about your illness. No one wants to frighten or upset their kids. But if you hide the truth, they'll probably figure out that something is wrong. Instead of letting your kids imagine the worst, let them know as much about what's happening as you think they can handle.

Reassure your children that it's not their fault, that cancer is not contagious, and that you're the same person you've always been.

If your children are adolescents, it may be even harder for them to cope with your diagnosis. Teenagers sometimes have difficulty showing their feelings, so you might not realize how upset they are. At a time when they're struggling to be independent, they may be unable to express how frightened they are that you're sick.

It's a good idea to ask your teenagers to help out from time to time. They'll appreciate being asked to take on some adult responsibilities. And they'll be comforted knowing they're helping you.

HELPING YOUR CHILDREN COPE

Try to maintain your children's regular routines as much as possible.

Make sure your children know they will be cared for, whatever the outcome.

If your kids are older, recognize their need for independence.

If behavioral problems, such as withdrawal or aggression, develop, seek professional guidance.

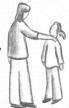

Making Financial Decisions

It's always a good time to dot the i's and cross the t's.

Financial planning is something everyone favors but not everyone acts on right away. If you've signed a will, a living will, and a healthcare proxy—essential documents for all adults to consider—you've already made some important long-term decisions. If those are things you, and perhaps your spouse or partner, have been putting off, there's no time like the present.

Just as you depend on your doctors and other healthcare professionals for advice in making the most appropriate treatment decisions, you'll probably want to turn to financial and legal experts for help with immediate and long-term planning. Often, the place to begin is with your lawyer, accountant, or financial adviser who will be able to work with you or recommend someone who specializes in this area.

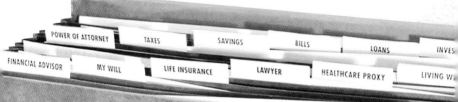

STEP ONE: GET YOUR RECORDS TOGETHER

If you know where all your financial, legal, and insurance documents are—and so does the person, or people, who might need access to them—you've already resolved one of the major problems family or friends may face when you're ill.

If things are scattered, or you keep track of the bills that have to be paid, and when they're due, in your head, you'll need to organize your paperwork. This is especially important if you're the person in charge of the day-to-day finances. You don't want an insurance policy to be cancelled or risk a tax delinquency because nobody knew a payment was due.

It might also be a good idea to consolidate savings and investment account statements, retirement plan documents, insurance policies, and outstanding loan notes in one place. If you keep electronic records, make sure to share password and user ID information.

If you don't have a joint checking account, and if there aren't two names on your safe deposit box, you may want to change that. If a family member or friend can write checks on your account, that person can keep the bills paid while you concentrate on recovery.

A DUAL ROLE FOR INSURANCE

You may want to investigate the terms of your life insurance contract. You may be able to draw on up to 90% of the value of your policy to pay healthcare costs. But you should get professional advice, preferably from an independent financial planner or fee-only insurance consultant, before taking this step. It will mean limited money is available for your survivors.

STEP TWO: FACING THE BIGGER ISSUES

You may have decided who should inherit your prized possessions. You may also have thought about your attitude toward life-extending treatments and who besides yourself you would want to authorize them. But your wishes might not be followed if you don't write them down in legally binding documents.

It's a good idea to talk to your lawyer about how you can ensure that your decisions are acted upon. Among the things he or she may recommend:

> ❝ *The human mind seems quite capable of planning for the worst and continuing to hope for the best.* ❞
>
> Robert Buckman, MD,
> *What You Really Need to Know About Cancer*

Review your will. Making a will and keeping it up-to-date is one of the most considerate and long-reaching things you can do for the people and institutions you love, whether or not you have cancer. You'll want to be sure that your bequests reflect your current wishes, and that, if you have minor children, you've named guardians. If you don't have a will, the court will probably follow a fairly rigid formula in disbursing your assets, and more of your estate may go to pay taxes than is necessary.

Consider a trust. You may want to use a trust to transfer assets to specific family members or friends and to direct how the money will be spent. If your goal is to give away your assets to qualify for Medicaid, a specific period of time—never less than three years—must pass between the time the trust is created and your application. However, you should always get legal advice before creating a trust to be sure it will accomplish your goals.

Sign a living will and healthcare proxy. A living will lets you specify the treatment you prefer if you're unable to make healthcare decisions on your own. If your wishes are not in writing, your family may not have the authority to choose what they believe you would want. You use the healthcare proxy to name the person whom you authorize to make your healthcare decisions if you are not able.

Investigate a power of attorney. You may want to give someone the legal right to handle your financial affairs by signing a power of attorney. Your lawyer can explain the reasons for signing such a document, the potential drawbacks, and the differences between ordinary, durable, and springing powers.

HANDLING THE PAPERWORK

You can ask your lawyer to prepare a power of attorney, will, living will, and healthcare proxy so you can sign them at the same time. Or you can use standard forms or software to prepare the documents, though you will probably want a lawyer to review them for accuracy. Remember, all of these documents—though not an irrevocable trust—can be revised or amended at any time.

TO LEARN MORE

Informed Decisions: The Complete Book of Cancer Diagnosis, Treatment, and Recovery
by Harmon J. Eyre, MD, Dianne Partie Lange, and Lois B. Morris, 2002

*F*or Primary Caregivers

When someone you love has cancer, your life changes too.

Cancer touches more people than those who are diagnosed with it. If your parent, spouse, child, or a close friend has cancer, you may find yourself their primary caregiver and supporter through treatment and recovery. While you're indispensable to them in many ways, one of the most important things you can do is encourage them to be as independent and self-sufficient as they want to be.

Playing Different Roles

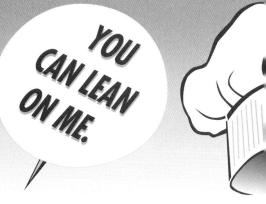

EMOTIONAL SUPPORT

DAILY ACTIVITIES

There are lots of different ways to be a caregiver. You'll provide emotional comfort. You may have to handle routine tasks like shopping or paying bills when the patient is having treatments or be ready to fill in at the last minute in a car pool or a committee meeting. You may schedule appointments and take the patient to them. You may act as a patient advocate, working with doctors, nurses, and the insurance company to get the best care for your loved one.

At the same time, while you might find yourself taking over a lot of your loved one's responsibilities, it's important to remember that the more control they have over their own lives, the better. If they are able to perform certain chores or tasks without your assistance, let them do it. They'll feel less frustrated and helpless.

CAREGIVER AND ADVOCATE
One of the best ways to be an effective caregiver is to learn all you can about your loved one's particular kind of cancer. Your local library, the American Cancer Society, and medical sites on the Internet are all great places to learn about the newest, most effective treatments and the facilities that offer them.

You may serve as a sounding board if the patient is struggling with choosing the best course of action. The doctors may try to enlist your support for the treatment they prefer. But you must be prepared to have your preferences and even professional recommendations ignored.

It's important to respect the choices a patient makes about his or her care. Although you may not agree, your loved one may have strong feelings about what's best. In that case, your role may be to provide access to accurate information about the illness and the treatment options available.

> **❝** When I learned I had cancer, I thought it was the end of the world, but it was merely an introduction to a whole new world. I quickly learned how much others could care, could give love, and could give of themselves. **❞**
>
> Martin Berkofsky, cancer survivor

HANDLING YOUR FINANCES

For most caregivers, one of the biggest responsibilities, after caring for your loved one, is managing the financial details of cancer treatment.

The hospital social worker is a good person to turn to for financial advice and assistance. It also makes sense to build a relationship with the insurance company caseworker assigned to the patient. For example, your plan may cover home nursing care.

> **TO LEARN MORE**
> *www.nfcacares.org*
> National Family Caregivers Association website

You might need to commit lots of your time to caring for the patient. If you need to take time off from work, federal law may protect your job during periods of unpaid family medical leave. Ask human resources about your employer's leave policy, and don't hesitate to press your case.

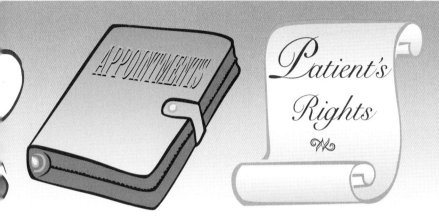

MANAGING APPOINTMENTS

PATIENT ADVOCACY

Take Care of Yourself

When you're taking care of someone else, you may focus exclusively on his or her health. But you'll be doing both of you a favor if you pay attention to your own health and happiness as well.

Make time for yourself. Try not to let illness be the only thing in your life. Get regular exercise, stay involved in your favorite activities, and plan time for fun.

Accept help. While you may feel like you're expected to do everything 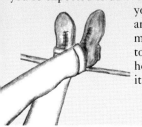 yourself—and you may want to—accept help when it's offered.

Let other family and friends handle some meals, for example, or fill in for you when you have errands to do.

Know your limitations. It's important to recognize that a patient may require more experienced care than you can provide. It can be hard to give up responsibility, but at times it's the best choice. Consult with the patient's doctor to determine when professional nursing services are warranted.

Let yourself be human. All kinds of feelings are normal. Just like the person you're taking care of, you'll have good days and bad days. It's okay to sometimes feel angry and frustrated that cancer has interrupted your lives and to wish you could get back to normal. Your emotions are natural, and you shouldn't ignore them or feel guilty. Instead, take a break, talk about your feelings with a friend, and realize what a great job you're doing.

For Supporters

Make a big difference with the little things you do.

When someone you know has cancer, there's a lot you can do, even though you're not the primary caregiver. Maybe you don't know where to begin, or you're worried that you'll say the wrong thing. Most people with cancer, however, are glad to know that their friends and extended family are still part of their lives. If you're willing, you're in a position to provide a lot of comfort and another motivation to get well.

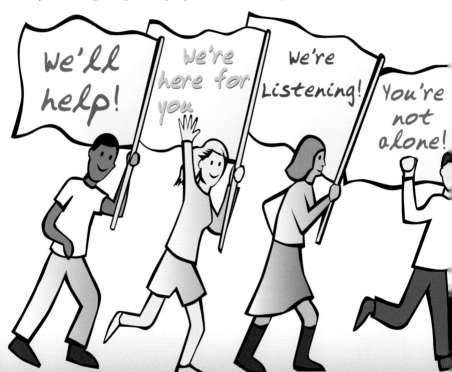

LEARNING TO LISTEN

One of the most caring ways to help is through conversation. Even if you feel awkward talking about illness, following a few simple guidelines can make it easier:

Listen. People who've been diagnosed with cancer face a lot of fear and uncertainty. Sometimes what your friend or family member needs most is someone who'll listen to what he or she is going through. You don't need to have answers, just a sympathetic ear.

Be sensitive to the patient's feelings. When a friend or family member has cancer, your first instinct may be to say that everything will be all right. But lots of people undergoing treatment don't know how things will turn out. By trying to reassure your loved one, he or she may feel that you're dismissing legitimate complaints or fears. It's good to be optimistic, but don't forget that it's natural for someone with cancer to be upset and afraid.

Follow the patient's cue. One of the best ways to be a listener is to be sensitive to what the other person wants to talk about. It may be experiences you've shared in the past or plans for the future. But cancer patients may want—or need—to concentrate on their illness. Be willing to talk about anything that they want to talk about.

TO LEARN MORE
www.cancer.org
American Cancer Society website

CHANGED RELATIONSHIPS

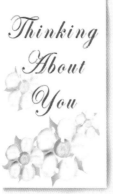

There may be times when your friend or family member doesn't feel like having company. Some people may not have the energy for visitors, and might be self-conscious about their appearance, which can change during treatment. Dealing with cancer can also be very time consuming, and your loved one might not have time to spend with you. Don't think that you're not a valued friend, or that there's nothing you can do. Sending cards or small gifts is a non-intrusive way to show your support until the person is ready for visits again.

HELPING THE CAREGIVER

You may be just as important to the patient's primary caregiver as you are to the patient. It's easy to admire the patience and endurance of the person who is in charge of another's healthcare. It's at least as important to provide them with an occasional respite.

One thing you can do is volunteer to stay with the patient on a regular schedule or drive him or her to appointments. Or you might do the shopping.

But you might also think of taking the caregiver to lunch, or to a movie, or sending that person flowers or a personal gift. While a caregiver may not expect to be pampered, your thoughtfulness and practical support will be appreciated.

The same things that apply to interacting with the patient—being willing to listen and encouraging them to choose the subject—will help the caregiver, too.

PRACTICAL HELP

Providing practical assistance is another important way to help a friend with cancer. Figure out what you're best at—maybe you're a great cook, or you have experience dealing with insurance companies. Here are some ideas:

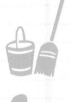

Make a dinner for the family. A homemade casserole can be put in the freezer and used when they need it.

Help do laundry or clean the house. Patients and their caregivers are often too busy or tired to take care of household chores.

Offer to take the children to a park or the movies for an afternoon. A fun outing for the kids can also be a mini-vacation for the parents.

Go to the library or check on the Internet to find the best hospitals that offer the latest cancer treatments.

Organize a fund-raiser to pay for part of the treatment that insurance might not cover. You can turn to friends, family, and local organizations like a religious community for contributions and support.

YOU CAN HELP

> *Typically, our loved ones are looking for something 'big' to do, but little things often mean the most. The smile on a friend's face who just stopped by to say 'Hi'. The sound of laughter filling a room full of friends or family. Or just some regular conversation and a little gossip to provide a welcome change. These are the little things anyone can do and be a hero.*
>
> Connie Payton
> *Stronger Than Cancer*

Glossary

Acupuncture: the ancient Eastern practice of inserting needles into the body at strategic points to redirect the flow of energy and relieve symptoms

Acute pain: sharp discomfort of short duration

Adenocarcinoma: carcinoma formed in the cells covering a gland

Adjuvant therapy: an additional therapy used to enhance the effectiveness of the primary therapy

Alternative therapy: a therapy outside the realm of conventional Western medicine that is used instead of **conventional** treatment

Analgesic: pain-fighting medication

Antibodies: proteins in the immune system that recognize antigens and create an immunity in response to them

Antigens: enzymes, toxins, and other substances that cause an immune response

Aromatherapy: the use of natural fragrances to promote physical and psychological wellbeing

Biopsy: the surgical removal of tissue for the purpose of diagnosis

Bone marrow: spongy material inside your bones where new blood cells are made

Bone marrow transplant (BMT) or stem cell transplant (SCT): the infusion of healthy stem cells to restore the immune system after a course of high-dose chemotherapy. In an **allogeneic** transplant, the patient receives cells from a donor. In an **autologous** transplant, the patient's own cells are reintroduced after they have been treated.

Botanical medicine: the use of plants to treat illness

Brachytherapy: the implantation of radioactive pellets, seeds, or wires to treat cancer

Cancer: group of diseases characterized by uncontrolled and invasive cell reproduction

Cancer centers: hospitals or clinics dedicated exclusively to treating cancer

Carcinoma: tumor formed in the cells that cover the skin and line the internal surfaces of the body

Chemotherapy: the treatment of cancer with drugs

Chronic pain: dull, long-lasting discomfort

Cold therapy: the medical use of cold temperatures, also called **cryotherapy**

Combination or multimodality treatment: the use of two or more conventional cancer treatments

Community hospitals: local private or public facilities that offer care for all illnesses in a community

Complementary and alternative medicine (CAM): any medical treatment that falls outside the scope of **conventional** Western medicine, such as **naturopathic medicine, nutritional therapy**, and **mind-body medicine**

Complementary therapy: a therapy outside the realm of conventional Western medicine that is used in addition to **conventional** treatment

Conventional therapy: a cancer treatment that is part of Western medical science and practice, such as **chemotherapy, radiation, surgery, immunotherapy**, or **stem cell transplant**

Cruciferous vegetables: the cabbage family of plants, including broccoli and cauliflower

Curative: to cure or remove the source of disease

Debulking: to remove part of a tumor, also called **cytoreductive**

Diagnostic: to evaluate the presence and extent of disease

Diarrhea: loose, watery stool

Dosimetrist: member of a radiation oncology team who calculates the dosage of radiation

Eastern medicine: the group of ancient medical systems developed in Asia, including traditional Chinese medicine (TCM) and ayurveda

Endoscopy: the use of a small camera to visually examine the inside of the body

External beam radiation therapy (EBRT): the use of radiation from an external source to penetrate the body and treat cancer

Fatigue: extreme tiredness and lack of energy

Fractionated dose chemotherapy: the administration of chemotherapy in small doses over a period of days, instead of in one large single dose, to improve effectiveness and reduce side effects

Grade: a measure, from one to four, of the degree of abnormality of cancer cells in comparison with normal cells. Lower grade cancer cells more closely resemble normal cells than high-grade cells.

Heat therapy: the medical use of high temperatures, also called **hyperthermia**

Hematologic: relating to the blood

Hematopoietic growth factor: immune substance that stimulates the growth of new blood cells

High dose rate brachytherapy: the delivery of internal radiation at a high dose over a short period of time

HLA (human leukocyte antigen) typing: genetic matching process used to determine bone marrow compatibility

Holistic: treating all aspects of a person's health, including physical, psychological, emotional, and spiritual aspects

Home care: medical therapy received in the patient's home

Homeopathy: the practice of using minuscule doses of natural substances to treat illness

Hormone therapy: treatments that block the effects of hormones on the body

Hospice care: end-of-life treatment that focuses on relieving symptoms, maintaining quality of life, and preserving dignity rather than curing illness

Hospice center: a residential option for those who want to receive hospice care

Hyperthermia: the use of high temperatures to destroy cancer cells

Hypnosis: a relaxed, sleep-like state of consciousness during which the patient is responsive to suggestion

Immunologist: a doctor who specializes in treating cancer with medications that reinforce the immune system

Immunotherapy: the use of medication to reinforce the immune system, also called **biological therapy** or **biological response modifier therapy**

Integrative cancer care facility: a hospital or clinic that treats cancer with both conventional and complementary therapies

Intensity modulated radiation therapy (IMRT): the use of computer imaging to deliver thousands of precisely shaped beams of external radiation that conform to the contours of the tumor

Interferons: immune system proteins that make cancer easier for your immune cells to recognize

Interleukins: hormone-like substances that stimulate the growth of white blood cells

Intra-arterial chemotherapy: the delivery of cancer drugs through an artery directly to the site of a tumor

Intraperitoneal chemotherapy: the delivery of chemotherapy directly to the peritoneal cavity in the abdomen to treat ovarian cancer

Leukemia: cancer of the blood or blood-forming organs

Liposarcoma: cancer of fatty tissue

Local therapy: a therapy that affects one part or region of the body

Lumpectomy: the surgical removal of a breast tumor, while preserving as much of the normal breast tissue as possible

Lymphatic system: the network of nodes and vessels that circulates lymph fluid

Lymphedema: a build-up of lymph fluid that causes swelling

Lymph fluid: the fluid that carries immune system cells throughout the body

Lymphoma: cancer of the lymphatic system

Mammosite® radiation therapy (MRT): the use of brachytherapy from within the site of a lumpectomy to destroy remaining cancerous cells

Massage therapy: the manipulation of muscles to promote relaxation and relieve pain

Medicaid: state sponsored healthcare for low-income families

Medical oncologist: a doctor who specializes in treating cancer with chemotherapy

Medicare: federal government sponsored healthcare for those who are 65 or older or who are permanently disabled

Meditation: Eastern spiritual practice that can be used therapeutically to promote relaxation and mental focus

Metastasis: the spread of cancerous cells through the lymph system to other sites in the body

Mind-Body medicine: the system of treatments designed to help the mind strengthen the immune system, also called **Psychoneuroimmunology (PNI)**

Monoclonal antibodies: immune system cells that are engineered to fight a specific tumor

Natural medicine: the treatment of illness using natural and non-toxic remedies

Nausea: a feeling of upset stomach or the desire to vomit

NED (no evidence of disease): when cancer is undetectable, although some cells may remain

Neo-adjuvant therapy: therapy used before primary therapy

Nerve surgery: the injection of medication or the severing of nerves to block pain

Non-myeloablative transplant: a less toxic approach to stem cell transplant using lower doses of chemotherapy, sometimes called a **mini-transplant**

Nutrition: the study of the effect of diet and nutrients on health and illness

Occupational therapy: working with a healthcare professional to overcome any physical side effects of treatment and to maintain independence in daily life

Osteosarcoma: cancer of the bone

Palliative: to relieve cancer-related symptoms

Passive exercise: the manipulation of a person's limbs by a physical therapist to improve flexibility and circulation

Pathologist: a doctor who examines and tests tissue to diagnose disease

Photodynamic therapy: the use of non-toxic, photosensitizing agents to make cancer cells vulnerable to laser treatment

Physical medicine: the use of stretches, exercise, and other physical therapies to treat illness and injury

Physical therapy: the use of exercise, massage, and other treatments to improve movement and promote healing

Preventive: inhibits or prevents the development of disease

Primary therapy: the main therapy used to treat cancer

Primary tumor: initial site of cancerous growth

Private hospital: a hospital that is owned by a company or individuals rather than the government

Prostate specific antigen (PSA): a protein created by the prostate gland that can be used as a tumor marker for prostate cancer

Prosthesis: the replacement of a missing part of the body with an artificial substitute

Psychiatrist: a medical physician who specializes in helping people overcome depression and other psychological challenges with counseling, medication, and other therapies

Psychology: the study of the mind and its influence on behavior

Psychoneuroimmunology (PNI): the study of the relationship between the mind and the immune system, also called **mind-body medicine**

Public hospital: a hospital supported by government funds

Qi gong: the Chinese meditative practice that uses **visualization** and gentle movement to promote wellness

Radiation oncologist: a doctor who specializes in treating cancer with radiation therapy

Radiation physicist: an expert in the field of radiation, in charge of maintaining the radiation therapy equipment

Radiation therapist: the operator of radiation therapy equipment

Radiation therapy: the treatment of cancer with high-energy waves

Radiation therapy nurse: a nurse with expertise in caring for patients who are undergoing radiation therapy

Radiofrequency ablation: the use of electrical energy to destroy cancer cells

Reconstructive: to rebuild tissue or restore appearance

Regional hospitals: large private or public facilities that offer care for all illnesses

Reiki: the Japanese practice of transferring energy from a practitioner to a patient through the hands

Remission: when diagnostic tests find no evidence of cancer

Resistive bands: lengths of stretchy rubber used to rebuild muscle and promote flexibility

Sarcoma: cancer formed in the connective tissue

Scans: cross-sectional x-rays of internal organs generated with a computer

Sentinel lymph node mapping and biopsy: the use of radioactive dyes to identify and examine the nodes to which a cancer is likely to spread, for diagnostic purposes

Skin irritation: rash, redness, itching, or burning, caused by irritation of the skin

Social worker: a professionally trained counselor who promotes the welfare and wellbeing of individuals. Most social workers hold an undergraduate or graduate degree in the discipline

Spiritual counseling: comfort and guidance on religious and spiritual matters

Squamous cell carcinoma: carcinoma formed from the flat cells covering non-glandular surfaces

Stage: a measure of whether and how far cancer has advanced

Staging: to determine the stage of cancer

State insurance commissioner: official in state government responsible for regulating insurance companies and investigating consumer insurance complaints

Stem cells: immature cells that have the ability to develop into a specific kind of cell, such as red and white blood cells and platelets

Surgery: treating disease or symptoms by removing tissue

Surgical oncologist: a doctor who specializes in using surgery to treat cancer

Systemic therapy: a therapy that treats or affects the entire body

Tai chi: the Chinese practice of slow, meditative movement

Tamoxifen: a drug used to block the effect of estrogen on hormone-responsive cancers

TENS (transcutaneous electrical nerve stimulation): the use of electric currents to disrupt nerve signals and reduce pain

3-D conformal radiation: the use of multiple beams of radiation that have been computer-designed to target a tumor

TNM: measurement of the **tumor,** cancerous **lymph nodes,** and **metastases,** used to determine a cancer's stage

Traditional Chinese medicine (TCM): the ancient system of medicine developed in China and based on the presence of energy known as *Qi,* translated as "life force"

Tumor marker: substance in the blood that can indicate the presence of cancer

Ultrasonic surgical aspiration: the use of sound waves to break a tumor into small pieces that are then removed by vacuum

University medical center: a hospital associated with a medical school

Visualization: the use of mental imagery and imagination to affect physical processes and focus the mind on healing

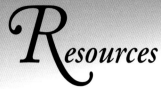

Resources

The following is a list of organizations, websites, and books that you may find helpful as you seek support and information. This list is not comprehensive and does not constitute an endorsement of these groups.

GENERAL INFORMATION

American Cancer Society (ACS)
National Home Office
1599 Clifton Road, NE
Atlanta, GA 30329-4251
www.cancer.org
Toll-free: 1-800-ACS-2345
(1-800-227-2345)
The American Cancer Society has local offices across the country. The ACS offers educational materials about cancer, runs a variety of programs for patients and their families, and can direct you to services in your area.

National Cancer Institute (NCI)
NCI Public Inquiries Office
Suite 3036A
6116 Executive Boulevard, MSC8322
Bethesda, MD 20892-8322
www.cancer.gov
Toll-free: 1-800-4-CANCER
(1-800-422-6237)
The federal government's primary agency for cancer research, the NCI provides comprehensive and up-to-date information on cancer prevention, diagnosis, and treatment. To learn about clinical trials, visit the NCI website or call the toll-free number. The NCI also subsidizes a small number of state-of-the-art, comprehensive cancer centers that meet its criteria (listed at the back of this section).

Cancer Treatment Research Foundation
www.ctrf.org
This non-profit foundation funds research that advances the science of cancer treatments. The website offers information and support for cancer patients.

Medlineplus Health Information
www.nlm.nih.gov/medlineplus
A service of the US National Library of Medicine and the National Institutes of Health, this online resource provides listings of doctors and physicians, information on medications, a medical encyclopedia and dictionaries, and other resources. The site is updated daily.

Association of Cancer Online Resources
www.acor.org
This non-profit organization brings together state-of-the-art Web resources and mailing lists for patients and their families.

TYPES OF CANCER

BRAIN TUMORS
American Brain Tumor Association
2720 River Road
Des Plaines, IL 60018
www.abta.org
Toll-free: 1-800-886-2282

BREAST CANCER
National Alliance of Breast Cancer Organizations
9 East 37th Street, 10th Floor
New York, NY 10016
www.nabco.org
Toll-free: 1-888-80-NABCO
(1-888-806-2226)

The Susan G. Komen Breast Cancer Foundation
www.komen.org
Toll-free: 1-800-IM-AWARE
(1-800-462-9273)

Y-Me National Breast Cancer Organization
www.y-me.org
Toll-free: (English) 1-800-221-2141
(Spanish) 1-800-986-9505

COLORECTAL CANCERS
Colon Cancer Alliance, Inc.
175 Ninth Avenue
New York, NY 10011
www.ccalliance.org
Toll-free: 1-877-422-2030

Colorectal Cancer Network
PO Box 182
Kensington, MD 20895-0182
www.colorectal-cancer.net
1-301-879-1500

GYNECOLOGICAL CANCERS

National Cervical Cancer Coalition
www.nccc-online.org
Toll-free: 1-800-685-5531

HEAD AND NECK CANCER

Let's Face It USA
www.faceit.org
1-360-676-7325

HEMATOLOGIC CANCER

International Myeloma Foundation
www.myeloma.org
Toll-free: 1-800-452-CURE
(1-800-452-2873)

The Leukemia and Lymphoma Society
Home Office
1311 Mamaroneck Avenue
White Plains, NY 10605
www.leukemia-lymphoma.org/hm_lls
1-914-949-5213

Lymphoma Research Foundation of America
www.lymphoma.org
Toll-free: 1-800-500-9976

KIDNEY CANCER

The Kidney Cancer Association
www.nkca.org
Toll-free: 1-800-850-9132

LUNG CANCER

American Lung Association
www.lungusa.org
Toll-free: 1-800-LUNG-USA
(1-800-586-4872)

PROSTATE CANCER

Association for the Cure of Cancer of the Prostate
www.capcure.org
Toll-free: 1-800-757-CURE
(1-800-757-2873)

SKIN CANCER

The Skin Cancer Foundation
www.skincancer.org
Toll-free: 1-800-SKIN-490
(1-800-754-6490)

COMPLEMENTARY THERAPIES

American Association of Naturopathic Physicians (AANP)
www.naturopathic.org
The AANP can help you find a qualified ND in your area.

American Institute for Cancer Research (AICR)
www.aicr.org
Toll-free: 1-800-843-8114

The AICR supports research and public education about the relationship between nutrition and cancer.

National Cancer Institute (NCI)
www.nci.nih.gov/cancerinfo/treatment/cam
The NCI website presents new research about the use of CAM therapies in the treatment of cancer.

National Center for Complementary and Alternative Medicine
www.nccam.nih.gov
Toll-free: 1-888-644-6226
International: 1-301-519-3153
For hearing impaired: 1-866-464-3615
This agency of the National Institutes of Health offers information, research, resources, and advisories on the use of complementary and alternative therapies to treat disease.

CONVENTIONAL TREATMENT

BONE MARROW TRANSPLANT

The National Marrow Donor Program (NMDP)
www.marrow.org
Toll-free: 1-800-MARROW2
(1-800-627-7692)
Office of Patient Advocacy (OPA):
Toll-free: 1-888-999-6743
This non-profit organization matches unrelated donors and patients. Its patient advocacy office also provides information about insurance coverage and medical facilities.

IMMUNOTHERAPY

Cancer Research Institute (CRI)
www.cancerresearch.org
The CRI funds research on immunotherapy, provides educational resources, and can help locate clinical trials.

FINANCIAL AND LEGAL

CancerandCareers.org
www.cancerandcareers.org
This website, sponsored by Cosmetic Executive Women, is a resource and community for working women with cancer.

National Association of Insurance Commissioners
www.naic.org

Patient Advocate Foundation
www.patientadvocate.org
Toll-free: 1-800-532-5274
   This national, non-profit group helps patients resolve disputes with their insurers and handle financial and professional issues.

HOSPICE CARE

Hospice Foundation of America
www.hospicefoundation.org
   This organization offers resources, information, and support for those interested in hospice care.

National Hospice and Palliative Care Organization
www.nhpco.org
   This site offers information on hospice care and a searchable database of hospice care providers.

SUPPORT

Cancer Care, Inc.
www.cancercare.org
Toll-free: 1-800-813-HOPE
(1-800-813-4673)
   This non-profit organization has a hotline and website offering education, counseling, and practical assistance.

Gilda's Club
www.gildasclub.org
   Named in honor of comedian Gilda Radner, Gilda's Club provides information and resources for people living with cancer.

SYMPTOMS AND SIDE EFFECTS

Oncology Nursing Society
www.cancersymptoms.org
   The Oncology Nursing Society's website offers comprehensive information about cancer pain.

BOOKS

Choices: The New, Most Up-to-Date Sourcebook for Cancer Information by Marion Morra and Eve Potts. Avon Books, 1994.

Choices in Healing: Integrating the Best of Conventional and Complementary Approaches to Cancer by Michael Lerner. MIT Press, 1996.

Comprehensive Cancer Care: Integrating Alternative, Complementary, and Conventional Therapies by James S. Gordon, MD, and Sharon Curtin. Perseus, 2000.

Everyone's Guide to Cancer Therapy: How Cancer is Diagnosed, Treated, and Managed Day to Day by Malin Dollinger, MD, Ernest H. Rosenbaum, MD, and Greg Cable. Somerville House, 1997.

Informed Decisions: The Complete Book of Cancer Diagnosis, Treatment, and Recovery by Harmon J. Eyre, MD, Dianne Partie Lange, and Lois B. Morris. American Cancer Society, 2001.

The Chemotherapy & Radiation Therapy Survival Guide: Information, Suggestions, and Support to Help You Get Through Treatment by Judith McKay, RN, OCN, and Nancee Hirano, RN, MS, AOCN. New Harbinger Publications, 1998.

The Complete Cancer Survival Guide by Peter Teeley and Philip Bashe. Doubleday, 2000.

The Force Program: The Proven Way to Fight Cancer Through Physical Activity by Jeff Berman, Fran Fleegler, MD, and John Hanc. Ballantine, 2001.

What You Really Need to Know About Cancer: A Comprehensive Guide for Patients and Their Families by Robert Buckman, MD. Johns Hopkins University Press, 1997.

BOOKS BY CTCA AUTHORS

Beating Cancer with Nutrition by Patrick Quillin, PhD, RD, CNS, and Noreen Quillin. Nutrition Times Press, 2001.

Challenge Cancer and Win!: Step-by-Step Nutrition Action Plans for Your Specific Cancer by Kim Dalzell, PhD, RD, LD. Nutriquest, 2002.

How to Prevent and Treat Cancer with Natural Medicine by Michael Murray, ND, Tim Birdsall, ND, Joseph E. Pizzorno, ND, and Paul Reilly, ND. Riverhead Books, 2002.

Stronger than Cancer by Connie Payton. Compendium, 2002.

There's No Place Like Hope: A Guide to Beating Cancer in Mind-Sized Bites by Vickie Girard. Compendium, 2001.

TREATMENT FACILITIES

CANCER TREATMENT CENTERS OF AMERICA (CTCA)

CTCA Headquarters
3150 Salt Creek Lane, Suite 118
Arlington Heights, IL 60005
www.cancercenter.com
Toll-free: 1-800-FOR-HELP
(1-800-367-4357)

CTCA at Midwestern Regional Medical Center
2520 Elisha Avenue
Zion, IL 60099
Toll-free: 1-800-322-9183

CTCA at Southwestern Regional Medical Center
2408 East 81st Street
Tulsa, OK 74137
Toll-free: 1-800-788-0448

CTCA at Seattle Cancer Treatment and Wellness Center
122 16th Avenue East
Seattle, WA 98112
Toll-free: 1-800-321-9272

CTCA at Hampton Roads
335 Crawford Street
Portsmouth, VA 23704
Toll-free: 1-800-615-3055

NATIONAL CANCER INSTITUTE COMPREHENSIVE CANCER CENTERS

ALABAMA
University of Alabama at Birmingham Comprehensive Cancer Center
1824 Sixth Avenue South
Birmingham, AL 35924-3300
www.ccc.uab.edu
Toll-free: 1-800-UAB-0933
(1-800-822-0933)

ARIZONA
Arizona Cancer Center
The University of Arizona
1515 North Campbell Avenue
PO Box 245024
Tucson, AZ 85724
www.azcc.arizona.edu
Toll-free: 1-800-622-COPE
(1-800-622-2673)
Email: copeline@azcc.arizona.edu

Mayo Clinic Cancer Center—Scottsdale
13400 East Shea Boulevard
Scottsdale, AZ 85259
www.MayoClinic.org/scottsdale
1-480-301-8000

CALIFORNIA
Chao Family Comprehensive Cancer Center
University of California at Irvine
101 The City Drive
Building 23, Route 81
Orange, CA 92868
www.ucihs.uci.edu/cancer
1-714-456-8200

City of Hope
Cancer Center and Beckman Research Institute
1500 East Duarte Road
Duarte, CA 91010
www.cityofhope.org
Toll-free: 1-800-826-HOPE
(1-800-826-4673)

Jonsson Comprehensive Cancer Center at UCLA
8-684 Factor Building
UCLA Box 951781
Los Angeles, CA 90095-1781
www.cancer.mednet.ucla.edu
1-381-825-5268
Email: JcccInfo@mednet.ucla.edu

University of California, San Diego Cancer Center
9500 Gilman Drive
La Jolla, CA 92093-0658
www.cancer.ucsd.edu
1-858-534-7600

University of California, San Francisco Comprehensive Cancer Center
Box 0128, UCSF, 2340 Sutter Street
San Francisco, CA 94143-0128
www.cc.ucsf.edu
Toll-free: 1-800-888-8664
Email: cceditor@cc.ucsf.edu

USC/Norris Comprehensive Cancer Center and Hospital
1441 Eastlake Avenue
Los Angeles, CA 90033-0804
www.ccnt.hsc.usc.edu
Toll-free: 1-800-USC-CARE
(1-800-872-2273)
Email: cainfo@ccnt.hsc.usc.edu

COLORADO
University of Colorado Cancer Center
Box F-704, 1665 North Ursula Street
Aurora, CO 80010
www.uccc.info
Toll-free: 1-800-621-7621

CONNECTICUT
Yale Cancer Center
Yale University School of Medicine
333 Cedar Street, PO Box 208028
New Haven, CT 06520-8028
www.med.yale.edu/ycc

DISTRICT OF COLUMBIA
Lombardi Cancer Center
Georgetown University
Medical Center
3800 Reservoir Road, NW
Washington, DC 20007
www.lombardi.georgetown.edu
1-202-784-4000

FLORIDA
**H. Lee Moffitt Cancer Center and
Research Institute at the University of
South Florida**
12902 Magnolia Drive
Tampa, FL 33612-9497
www.moffitt.usf.edu
Toll-free: 1-888-MOFFITT
(1-888-663-3488)

**Mayo Clinic Cancer Center—
Jacksonville**
4500 San Pablo Road,
Jacksonville, FL 32224
www.MayoClinic.org/jacksonville
1-904-953-2000

ILLINOIS
**The Robert H. Lurie
Comprehensive Cancer Center of
Northwestern University**
Olson Pavilion 8250
303 East Chicago Avenue
Chicago, IL 60611
www.cancer.northwestern.edu
1-312-908-5250

IOWA
**The Holden Comprehensive Cancer
Center at the University of Iowa**
5970-Z JPP, 200 Hawkins Drive
Iowa City, IA 52242-1009
www.uihealthcare.com/
DeptsClinicalServices/CancerCenter
Toll-free: 1-800-777-8442

MARYLAND
**The Johns Hopkins Oncology Center
Weinberg Building**
401 North Broadway
Baltimore, MD 21231-2410
www.hopkinskimmelcancercenter.org
For patient referral: 1-410-955-8964

MASSACHUSETTS
Dana-Farber Cancer Institute
44 Binney Street
Boston, MA 02155
www.dana-farber.org
Toll-free: 1-866-408-DFCI
(1-866-408-3324)

MICHIGAN
**Barbara Ann Karmanos
Cancer Institute**
Wertz Clinical Center

4100 John R
Detroit, MI 48201
www.karmanos.org
Toll-free: 1-800-KARMANOS
(1-800-527-6267)
Email: info@karmanos.org

**University of Michigan Comprehensive
Cancer Center**
1500 East Medical Center Drive
CCGC 6-303
Ann Arbor, MI 48109-0944
www.cancer.med.umich.edu
Toll-free: 1-800-865-1125
Email: wwwcancer@umich.edu

MINNESOTA
Mayo Clinic Cancer Center
200 First Street, SW
Rochester, MN 55905
www.MayoClinic.org/rochester
1-507-284-2511

University of Minnesota Cancer Center
Mayo Mail Code 806
420 Delaware Street, SE
Minneapolis, MN 55455
www.cancer.umn.edu
1-612-624-8484
Email: info@cancer.umn.edu

NEW HAMPSHIRE
Norris Cotton Cancer Center
Dartmouth-Hitchcock Medical Center
One Medical Center Drive
Lebanon, NH 03756
www.dartmouth.edu/dms/nccc
Toll-free: 1-800-639-6918
Email: cancerhelp@dartmouth.edu

NEW JERSEY
The Cancer Institute of New Jersey
195 Little Albany Street
New Brunswick, NJ 08901
http://cinj.umdnj.edu
1-732-235-CINJ (1-732-235-2465)

NEW YORK
**Herbert Irving Comprehensive
Cancer Center**
Columbia Presbyterian Center
New York-Presbyterian Hospital
PH 18, Room 200
622 West 168th Street
New York, NY 10032
www.ccc.columbia.edu
1-212-305-9327

Kaplan Comprehensive Cancer Center
New York University School of
Medicine
550 First Avenue
New York, NY 10016
www.nyucancerinstitute.org
1-212-263-6485

Memorial Sloan-Kettering Cancer Center
1275 York Avenue
New York, NY 10021
Toll-free: 1-800-525-2225
www.mskcc.org

Roswell Park Cancer Institute
Elm and Carlton Streets
Buffalo, NY 14263-0001
www.roswellpark.org
Toll-free: 1-877-ASK-RPCI
(1-877-275-7724)

NORTH CAROLINA
Comprehensive Cancer Center of Wake Forest University
Wake Forest University
Baptist Medical Center
Medical Center Boulevard
Winston-Salem, NC 27157
www.bgsm.edu/cancer
Toll-free: 1-800-446-2255

Duke Comprehensive Cancer Center
Duke University Medical Center
301 MSRB DUMC Box 3843
Durham, NC 27710
www.cancer.duke.edu
Toll-free: 1-888-ASK-DUKE
(1-888-275-3853)

UNC Lineberger Comprehensive Cancer Center
School of Medicine
University of North Carolina at
Chapel Hill Campus Box 7295
Chapel Hill, NC 27599-7295
http://cancer.med.unc.edu
1-919-966-3036

OHIO
Ireland Cancer Center
11100 Euclid Avenue
Cleveland, OH 44106
www.irelandcancercenter.org
Toll-free: 1-800-641-2422
Email: info@irelandcancercenter.org

The Ohio State University Comprehensive Cancer Center
The James Cancer Hospital and
Solove Research Institute
300 West 10th Avenue, Suite 519
Columbus, OH 43210
www.jamesline.com
Toll-free: 1-800-293-5066
Email: cancerinfo@jamesline.com

PENNSYLVANIA
Abramson Cancer Center of the University of Pennsylvania
15th Floor, Penn Tower
3400 Spruce Street-2 Donner
Philadelphia, PA 19104-4283

http://oncolink.upenn.edu
Toll-free: 1-800-789-PENN
(1-800-789-7366)

Fox Chase Cancer Center
7701 Burholme Avenue
Philadelphia, PA 19111
www.fccc.edu
Toll-free: 1-888-FOX CHASE
(1-888-369-2427)

University of Pittsburgh Cancer Institute
200 Lothrop Street
Pittsburgh, PA 15260
www.upci.upmc.edu
Toll-free: 1-800-237-4PCI
(1-800-237-4724)
Email: PCI-INFO@msx.upmc.edu

TENNESSEE
The Vanderbilt-Ingram Cancer Center
Vanderbilt University
691 Preston Building
Nashville, TN 37232-6838
www.vicc.org
Toll-free: 1-800-811-8480 (for clinical trial or treatment information)
1-888-488-4089 (for all other calls)

TEXAS
The University of Texas M.D. Anderson Cancer Center
1515 Holcombe Boulevard
Houston, TX 77030
www.mdanderson.org
Toll-free: 1-800-392-1611

VERMONT
Vermont Cancer Center
University of Vermont
Health Science Research Facility
149 Beaumont Avenue
Burlington, VT 05405
www.vermontcancer.org
1-802-656-4414
Email: vcc@uvm.edu

WASHINGTON
Fred Hutchinson Cancer Research Center
1100 Fairview Avenue North
PO Box 19024
Seattle, WA 98109-1024
www.fhcrc.org
Toll-free: 1-800-804-8824

WISCONSIN
University of Wisconsin Comprehensive Cancer Center
600 Highland Avenue, K5/601
Madison, WI 53792-6164
www.cancer.wisc.edu
Toll-free: 1-800-622-8922
E-mail: uwcc@uwcc.wisc.edu

*I*ndex